Praise for *Outsmarting Overeating*

"*Outsmarting Overeating* does more than offer a solid, step-by-step approach to building a healthy relationship with food and eating. It offers a thoughtful, compassionate, effective path for healing your life, emotions, and relationships. Highly recommended!"

— Donald Altman, MA, LPC, author of *One-Minute Mindfulness* and *Art of the Inner Meal*

"If you find that your relationship to food and eating is a problem and you want to find a way to change it without dieting, *Outsmarting Overeating* is sure to add some wonderful tools to your toolbox. Karen R. Koenig's newest book elevates the self-help genre to a whole new level of writing that will benefit every reader!"

— Megrette Fletcher, MEd, RD, CDE, cofounder of The Center for Mindful Eating and coauthor of *Eat What You Love, Love What You Eat with Diabetes*

"This is a nurturing, realistic system for developing healthy life skills and then applying them to eating behaviors."

— Anna Jedrziewski, *Retailing Insight*

Praise for Karen R. Koenig's Previous Books

"What [*The Rules of 'Normal' Eating*] offers is a perspective on working through some of the many misbeliefs and setbacks that prevent many of us from eating a 'normal' diet. Karen outlines what each rule would look like in real life, and gives practical advice for how to start to change lifelong habits into healthier ones."

— Rebecca Bitzer, The Nutrition Experts, EmpoweredEatingBlog.com

"Using humor, plain talk, examples from her clinical experi... tion exercises, case studies, and homew... know that their yo-yo patterns of eating... She shies away from easy answers and... crete actions to developing a *permanent,*

—...west *Book Review*

"Since women, at least those of us in the Western World, are socialized to be pleasers, Karen Koenig has written a wonderful book to help us save ourselves from ourselves....[*Nice Girls Finish Fat*] is deceptively simple and chock-full of stories to help readers see themselves in the lessons she teaches. She is a master clinician."

— Dr. Beth Erickson, author of *Marriage Isn't for Sissies*

"*What Every Therapist Needs to Know about Treating Eating and Weight Issues* is a wonderful tool for therapists to gain more insight on the occasional eating and weight problems in clients."

— *International Journal of Psychotherapy*

Outsmarting Overeating

Also by Karen R. Koenig

The Food and Feelings Workbook:
A Full Course Meal on Emotional Health

Nice Girls Finish Fat:
Put Yourself First and Change Your Eating Forever

The Rules of "Normal" Eating:
A Commonsense Approach for Dieters, Overeaters, Undereaters,
Emotional Eaters, and Everyone in Between!

Starting Monday:
Seven Keys to a Permanent, Positive Relationship with Food

What Every Therapist Needs to Know
about Treating Eating and Weight Issues

Outsmarting Overeating

BOOST YOUR LIFE SKILLS, END YOUR FOOD PROBLEMS

Karen R. Koenig, LCSW, MED

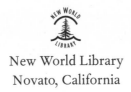

New World Library
Novato, California

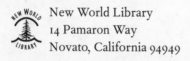

New World Library
14 Pamaron Way
Novato, California 94949

Text design by Tona Pearce Myers

Library of Congress Cataloging-in-Publication Data
Koenig, Karen R., date.
 Outsmarting overeating : boost your life skills, end your food problems / Karen R. Koenig, LCSW, MEd.
    pages   cm
Includes bibliographical references and index.
ISBN 978-1-60868-316-1 (paperback)
 1. Eating disorders—Psychological aspects. 2. Food—Psychological aspects.
I. Title.
RC552.E18K634 2014
616.85'26—dc23   2014034245

First printing, January 2015
ISBN 978-1-60868-316-1
Printed in Canada on 100% postconsumer-waste recycled paper

New World Library is proud to be a Gold Certified Environmentally Responsible Publisher. Publisher certification awarded by Green Press Initiative. www.greenpressinitiative.org

10   9   8   7   6   5   4   3   2   1

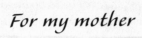

For my mother

Contents

Introduction

I bet you picked up this book with a groan of disbelief, thinking, here you are, *again*, reading *yet another* book to improve your eating habits. Perhaps you have been struggling for decades to make peace with the refrigerator and the scale. You forge a bit of progress, only to see it vanish into thin air as a crisis strikes or as you get fed up with working so darned hard to eat "normally." You may be sick to death of thinking about food — all the "shoulds" and "shouldn'ts," all the instructions telling you to "eat this" and "don't eat that" — that you're ready to throw up your hands in despair and accept your relationship with food, no matter how crummy it is.

Almost. The fact that you're reading these words means you still feel a spark of optimism — that maybe this book will turn your eating habits around once and for all, that it will tell you why you keep snacking when you're not hungry, eating past the point of being full, obsessing about food and weight, and choosing foods that endanger your health and happiness. So here you are, hoping against hope that this book will tell you how to put your eating problems behind you and leave them there.

It will! — because *Outsmarting Overeating* isn't a diet book. It's not even primarily about eating. It's about the rest of your life, the part that has been mucking up your relationship with food. Read on to discover the *real* reasons you have an eating problem and to learn a tried-and-true approach to putting food in its rightful place while simultaneously creating a better life for yourself.

During my three decades of working with troubled eaters, it's become glaringly obvious to me that a person's misguided relationship with food is a symptom of deeper, darker problems. The truth is, biology and heredity aside (and both can play a huge role in determining eating patterns and weight parameters), if you engage in unwanted, unhealthy eating with such frequency and ferocity that it ruins your self-esteem and damages your health, you're likely lacking a set of essential skills needed to better manage your life. Sure, you can benefit from nutritional information and behavioral techniques that will help you eat more healthfully. But you'll never succeed if the skills you use to cope with life's ups and downs are so weak and ineffective that eating has become your major strategy for facing your daily challenges, and if food is your greatest source of pleasure, most loved reward, most pursued passion, day's highlight, and bosom buddy.

Troubled eaters like you engage in mindless eating because that's the best way — the *only* way — you know how to get through the day, the week, the weekend, your life!

Though desperate to improve your relationship with food, you won't succeed merely by using the tired, old, well-meaning advice to count calories or fat grams, shop only the supermarket's perimeter, cut food portions way back, and weigh in daily. That's like expecting alcoholics to know how to deal with life without taking a drink, when they've always dealt with life by tossing down a few. Where, pray tell, would such know-how come from if alcohol has been keeping them afloat for years or decades? Where would it come from if food is the crutch you've been using to limp through life?

Attempts to eat better won't amount to a hill of beans unless you *also* possess essential skills to maneuver through life effectively and successfully — to beat the blahs and the blues, manage stress, achieve goals, establish and maintain functional relationships, take care of yourself physically and emotionally, think rationally, and create a passionate, meaningful life that makes you want to get out there and live rather than rent space in your refrigerator. Without new, effective strategies for being good to yourself and interacting with the world, you're condemned to old, destructive eating patterns no matter how grand your intentions or how strong your motivation. Without acquiring essential *life skills* that you lack, you're doomed to continue struggling with food and the scale and to remain unhappy, unhealthy, and unfulfilled.

What are life skills? According to the World Health Organization, they're "abilities for adaptive and positive behaviour that enable individuals to deal effectively with the demands and challenges of everyday life." Based on the list of skills that WHO developed, I've created a select skill set targeted specifically to troubled eaters. The life skills taught in this book are the same ones that I teach in my therapy and coaching sessions, my lectures and workshops, and I have touched on them in previous books. They are attitudes and actions that we're fortunate to learn in childhood. But many of us didn't learn them then because our parents taught us from their own, often dysfunctional, histories, distorted perspectives, limited knowledge base, and imperfect abilities.

Life skills are the missing piece of the eating-disorder puzzle and can be learned by anyone at any age. Bulletin: It's not just troubled eaters who need these skills; we *all* need them.

This book will teach them to you. Read on and you'll learn how to relax and let loose; soothe your ruffled emotions; sustain your motivation and achieve your goals; make effective decisions without driving yourself crazy before, while, and after you make them; create and maintain healthy relationships; find purpose and passion that suit your unique talents, interests, and abilities; and take such exquisite care of your body and mind that you wouldn't think of using food or inadequate self-care to harm them.

This book covers eight essential life skills, explaining the purpose of each one and giving examples to prove their necessity. It also illustrates how lacking each skill propels you toward unnecessary eating, and how, in turn, unwanted eating prevents skill development. For example, with poor problem-solving skills, you might raid the pantry at the first whisper that your company may start downsizing your department. Thrown into a panic, you may feel so overwhelmed and paralyzed that your brain stops working, while your desire for sweets and treats shifts into overdrive. And while you're chowing down, you're missing an opportunity to learn how to truly solve the problems posed by the possibility of losing your job.

Here are a few more examples. If you find your mind drifting back toward the past or zooming off into the future on a regular basis without your explicit permission, you may feel so full of regret or anxiety that you miss each marvelous moment of today. And, if you're not present when you're eating (or grocery shopping or preparing food), it's unlikely that you're going to attend to the task of feeding your body exactly what it wants in a quantity that suits it. By learning the skill of anchoring your mind to the present, you'll be able to consider the past or future consciously for specific reasons, then quickly recenter yourself in the here and now when you're eating or doing other activities.

If you've grown into an adult who believes she can't depend on people and tries to handle everything alone, you're at a distinct disadvantage when life gets rough-and-tumble, and your likelihood of turning to food for comfort and stabilization is good to excellent. When you're more skilled in trusting and depending on people — the right people, the ones who'll be there for you gladly and with wisdom — you'll find real comfort and security and won't even think about turning to food when you're in distress.

Here's a bit of information about the format of this book. Before you begin reading chapters, you'll find the "Life Skills Preassessment" questionnaire — a set of sixty questions to help you evaluate your life-skill strengths and weaknesses. At the end of the book, you'll find its companion, the "Life Skills Postassessment" questionnaire, which will show you the progress you've made and your remaining proficiency challenges.

Chapters include "Get Smart!" questions, which provide information about how you're doing with a particular life skill, help you identify barriers to gaining expertise, and teach you how to speed up skill acquisition. You'll also find "Skill Booster" activities at the end of every chapter, which will keep you practicing life skills between chapters.

After practicing these life skills for a while (okay, a *long* while), they'll become more automatic. You'll be less stressed, calmer, happier, centered, and well-balanced, as well as more competent to face life head-on. Once these skills are in place and have become part of your repertoire, you'll find them so powerful and effective for living your best life that food abuse will gradually become a distant memory. As author Maya Angelou succinctly puts it, "You did the best that you knew how. Now that you know better, you'll do better."

Life Skills Preassessment

---

*Life skills are abilities for adaptive and positive behaviour
that enable individuals to deal effectively with the demands
and challenges of everyday life.*

— World Health Organization

This questionnaire is designed to help you recognize your life-skill proficiencies and deficiencies — that is, to gauge strengths and weaknesses in managing life effectively and successfully. At the end of this book, you will find a Life Skills Postassessment that will help you determine what you've learned and which specific, challenging skill sets need more attention.

Although there are no right or wrong responses to the statements in this questionnaire, please give each one some thought before answering, and be honest. No judging yourself, puh-lease, if you're not as competent as you'd like to be. Instead of being hard on yourself, stay curious and maintain a mind-set that lets you know you'll feel a good deal better about your skills after doing the postassessment than you do right now. Remember, you're reading this book for self-knowledge that will help you permanently repair your relationship with food. And it will, I promise!

Instructions: Circle the number that best describes your response to each statement, with the number 1 representing *least true* and 10 representing *most true*.

1. Overall, I have effective life skills.

   1   2   3   4   5   6   7   8   9   10

2. I surround myself with people who have effective life skills.

   1   2   3   4   5   6   7   8   9   10

3. Improved life skills would help me eat "normally" and attain and maintain a healthy weight.

   1   2   3   4   5   6   7   8   9   10

4. I take excellent care of my health.

    1   2   3   4   5   6   7   8   9   10

5. I have routine medical tests, follow doctors' orders, and take care of emergency medical concerns right away.

    1   2   3   4   5   6   7   8   9   10

6. I get sufficient sleep most nights.

    1   2   3   4   5   6   7   8   9   10

7. I take vitamins and supplements or medication consistently.

    1   2   3   4   5   6   7   8   9   10

8. I get exercise (formal or informal) on a regular basis.

    1   2   3   4   5   6   7   8   9   10

9. I am generally in touch with and can identify my feelings.

    1   2   3   4   5   6   7   8   9   10

10. I value and am willing to experience all my feelings.

    1   2   3   4   5   6   7   8   9   10

11. Rather than judging them, I am curious about my feelings.

    1   2   3   4   5   6   7   8   9   10

12. I can tolerate intense and uncomfortable or conflicting feelings.

    1   2   3   4   5   6   7   8   9   10

13. I express emotions appropriately and effectively.

    1   2   3   4   5   6   7   8   9   10

14. I comfort and calm myself effectively.

    1   2   3   4   5   6   7   8   9   10

15. For the most part, I live consciously and in the present.

    1   2   3   4   5   6   7   8   9   10

16. I don't spend time unnecessarily worrying about the past.

    1   2   3   4   5   6   7   8   9   10

17. I don't spend time unnecessarily worrying about the future.

    1   2   3   4   5   6   7   8   9   10

18. I know that whatever befalls me in life, I will manage.

    1   2   3   4   5   6   7   8   9   10

19. I plan for the future, then let it take care of itself.

    1   2   3   4   5   6   7   8   9   10

20. I am comfortable in most social situations.

    1   2   3   4   5   6   7   8   9   10

21. I am generally honest and share my feelings with intimates.

    1   2   3   4   5   6   7   8   9   10

22. Intimates care about me as much as I care about them.

    1   2   3   4   5   6   7   8   9   10

23. I set boundaries with intimates, and they respect them.

    1   2   3   4   5   6   7   8   9   10

24. I take care of myself as well as I take care of others.

    1   2   3   4   5   6   7   8   9   10

25. I'm good at knowing who to trust and who not to trust.

    1   2   3   4   5   6   7   8   9   10

26. I know how to make and keep wonderful friends.

    1   2   3   4   5   6   7   8   9   10

27. I'm pretty even emotionally and avoid emotional extremes.

    1   2   3   4   5   6   7   8   9   10

28. I generally know when enough is enough.

    1   2   3   4   5   6   7   8   9   10

29. I don't tend to frequently overdo or underdo.

    1   2   3   4   5   6   7   8   9   10

30. I don't depend on others to regulate me emotionally.

   1   2   3   4   5   6   7   8   9   10

31. When I'm with difficult people, I stay on an even keel.

   1   2   3   4   5   6   7   8   9   10

32. I don't think in all-or-nothing, black-or-white terms.

   1   2   3   4   5   6   7   8   9   10

33. I value both structure and freedom.

   1   2   3   4   5   6   7   8   9   10

34. I'm skilled at troubleshooting and problem solving.

   1   2   3   4   5   6   7   8   9   10

35. I'm neither too cautious nor impulsive in decision making.

   1   2   3   4   5   6   7   8   9   10

36. I don't second-guess myself after making a decision.

   1   2   3   4   5   6   7   8   9   10

37. I don't put off decisions because they're hard to make.

   1   2   3   4   5   6   7   8   9   10

38. I have confidence in my critical-thinking skills.

   1   2   3   4   5   6   7   8   9   10

39. I generally reach my goals.

   1   2   3   4   5   6   7   8   9   10

40. I'm good at creating concrete, realistic goals for myself.

   1   2   3   4   5   6   7   8   9   10

41. I know how to divide big goals into smaller ones.

   1   2   3   4   5   6   7   8   9   10

42. I'm skilled at sustaining the effort needed to reach my goals.

   1   2   3   4   5   6   7   8   9   10

43. I'm good at maintaining my hard-won achievements.

   1   2   3   4   5   6   7   8   9   10

44. I don't sabotage my progress or achievements.

I   2   3   4   5   6   7   8   9   10

45. I recognize that all progress consists of baby steps.

I   2   3   4   5   6   7   8   9   10

46. My goals are composed of my wants, not "shoulds."

I   2   3   4   5   6   7   8   9   10

47. I can easily ask for or accept help in reaching my goals.

I   2   3   4   5   6   7   8   9   10

48. I always speak kindly to myself about myself.

I   2   3   4   5   6   7   8   9   10

49. I don't let other people be unkind or hurtful to me.

I   2   3   4   5   6   7   8   9   10

50. I don't have to be perfect.

I   2   3   4   5   6   7   8   9   10

51. I value myself and expect others to value me too.

I   2   3   4   5   6   7   8   9   10

52. I both love myself unconditionally and strive to do better.

I   2   3   4   5   6   7   8   9   10

53. I'm generally more curious about, than critical of, my mistakes.

I   2   3   4   5   6   7   8   9   10

54. I take failure in stride and learn from it.

I   2   3   4   5   6   7   8   9   10

55. I have a stable sense of myself.

I   2   3   4   5   6   7   8   9   10

56. I live a life balanced between obligations and play.

I   2   3   4   5   6   7   8   9   10

57. I can relax and let go fairly easily in healthy ways.

I   2   3   4   5   6   7   8   9   10

58. I know when I'm ready to work or play or relax.

    1   2   3   4   5   6   7   8   9   10

59. I rarely procrastinate or rebel against commitments.

    1   2   3   4   5   6   7   8   9   10

60. I live purposely and know the meaning of my life.

    1   2   3   4   5   6   7   8   9   10

CHAPTER I

The Definition and Purpose of Life Skills

Is Excelling at Cleaning My Plate a Life Skill?

You may think food is your main problem, but it isn't. Rather, food is the misguided *solution* to your real difficulties, and over the years misguided eating has morphed into a whopper unto itself. The truth is, your problem is that you never learned the skills and strategies everyone needs in order to live effectively and successfully. Think about it: you need skills for employment, relationships, parenting, and living in a community, for play and recreation, driving a car, and balancing your checkbook. No activity I can think of precludes having *some* degree of competence — not even tying your shoes!

So, agreed: everyone needs life skills? Of course, the bad news is that simply wishing for them won't make them magically appear. The good news is that these skills are learnable by anyone at any age at any time. We're *all* learning them to one degree or another as we muddle along, so join the crowd.

What are these must-have life skills? They're a set of universal competencies we all need to learn and practice to get the best out of life, rather than letting life get the best of us. Call them strategies or methods; tactics, tools, or techniques; competencies or abilities. What they boil down to are the essential maneuvers human beings must employ to engage with life successfully.

Specifically, here are the five basic life skills that span every culture, as identified by the World Health Organization's Department of Mental Health: (1) decision making and problem solving, (2) creative thinking and critical thinking, (3) communication and interpersonal skills, (4) self-awareness and empathy, and (5) coping with emotions and coping with stress.

I've taken the liberty of devising skill sets targeted to an audience of troubled eaters and focusing on the expertise they often lack regarding (1) wellness and physical self-care, (2) handling emotions, (3) living consciously, (4) building and maintaining relationships, (5) self-regulation, (6) problem solving and critical thinking, (7) setting and reaching goals, and (8) balancing work and play.

▰▰ Get Smart!

Do you still think you have only eating problems, or are you starting to recognize that your difficulties are due to not managing life all that well? Does that make you more, or less, optimistic about developing a positive, healthy relationship with food? Come up with a sentence that will put you in a positive frame of mind for reading this book and learning life skills.

What Are Essential Life Skills, and Where Do They Come From?

According to the 2003 *World Book Dictionary*, a skill is defined as an "ability gained by practice or knowledge; expertness." The most significant aspect of this definition is that a skill is something *gained by practice*. Like money, skills don't grow on trees, ready for you to pluck them off. Knowledge or expertise comes at the *end* of a process, not at the beginning, and life skills do not miraculously appear through wishin' and hopin' and thinkin' and prayin'. Unfortunately, many troubled eaters expect to excel at a task after one attempt or a few brief learning forays. Others believe that no matter how motivated they are and how much they practice, they'll never learn the skills others possess, because there's something inherently defective and unfixable about them.

The question of how life skills originate is complex. Certain talents and proclivities — art, music, math, language, dance, sports, writing, and so on — come to us through genetics. For example, I have two artist friends, one of whom is the son of a prolific portrait painter. The child of these two friends could, at eight years of age, outdraw and outpaint the adult me by a mile. We all know, or know of, families whose members shine in a particularly gifted way, and we generally accept that a certain amount of talent is innate. Alternatively, perfectly ordinary parents at times produce the most extraordinarily endowed children, and we wonder how *that* happened.

Although it's clear that heredity plays some role in our abilities, it's impossible to pinpoint how much is due to nature (genetics) and how much is due to nurture (socialization) — and I'm not here to debate or resolve the question. A useful way to think of the process is nature *via* nurture — that is, our environment helps us express the genetic tendencies with which we're born. In the end, we all have to make the best of what we bring into the world and how it's shaped by our personal history — by our parents, extended family, schooling, geography, social status, finances, race, ethnicity, gender, fortune and misfortune, culture, and other factors.

▰▰ Get Smart!

Take a look at my life-skills list and consider how your parents' skills stacked up. Can you see how you came to lack certain skills because of your upbringing? The idea is not to blame your parents (or yourself) but to understand how your deficits came to exist. It's a simple process of cause and effect. Remember, you didn't choose to miss out on learning essential life skills!

It would be naive to believe that life skills are learned on an even playing field. Obviously, if our parents were replete with these skills, especially those that improve a person's parenting abilities, we will be far better off than if they bumbled and stumbled through child rearing. Although I'm no sociologist, I can say from practicing psychology for more than thirty years, and from living on the planet for more than twice that long, that no particular race, gender, social class, ethnicity, or locale produces people with more effective life skills than any other.

Here's a case in point. When I was doing my first internship in social work, I worked with a lovely couple, both of whom had schizophrenia. In spite of their illness and living a substantial distance apart, these twenty-somethings were in love and seriously committed to each other. They both had low-level jobs, took their psychiatric medications consistently, attended therapy appointments regularly and on time (in spite of having to travel by public transportation in Boston), worked their tails off in sessions, and, in my presence at least, treated each other with respect and kindness. On the whole, although limited in some ways by mental illness, they had some pretty darned good life skills.

Compare this couple to psychiatrists who have sexual relations with their patients, to parents who charge onto the field where their child is playing a sport to berate a coach or an umpire, or to legislators shouting abuses at each other in the halls of Congress. Get my point? These examples show how people we believe *should* have better life skills very often don't. Moreover, I've met folks who had it fairly easy coming up who grew into adults with weak life skills, and survivors of the most egregious childhood abuses who manage their lives impressively by anyone's standards.

As far as I can ascertain, nothing inherent in anyone's upbringing is a surefire indicator that they're going to have stellar life skills. If I had to cite just one factor, however, it would be the life-skill level of a child's parents. What a boy or girl sees modeled at home goes a long way toward teaching him or her how to engage effectively with the world. Moreover, a child whose parents manage their own lives well will undoubtedly receive better treatment and socialization than a child whose parents' skill sets are spotty and ineffectual.

However, even that is not the whole story. Let's say a child grows up in a household in which her parents move from low-paying job to low-paying job, manage money poorly, drink or do illicit drugs regularly, scream at each other and their children, and mindlessly career through life, bouncing from one crisis to another. Does this automatically mean that their child is doomed to miss out on learning how to negotiate life? Not necessarily, if this child has a neighbor, teacher, or close relative who cares enough and has sufficient life skills to help shape the child's attitudes and behaviors. Sometimes, all a child needs is one caring, competent person, called a mentor, to make the difference between growing up with or without effective skills. Of course, the longer that children blunder through life without observing or being taught appropriate ways of managing it, the harder it will be to reverse their habits. Hard, mind you, but never impossible.

▰▰ Get Smart!

Aside from your parents, where else did you learn life skills as a child: from your favorite TV shows, books, movies, your best friend's parents, your parents' best friends, your teachers, relatives, a coach, or a religious leader?

Sometimes a child doesn't even need a real person to be guided in the right direction. A book, movie, TV series, or other story might spark an interest in or model acting appropriately. Here's a case in point. As a preteen, I angered fairly easily. Not that I had a wicked temper, but my low-grade irritation often leaked out in inappropriate ways. Then, I read *Little Women* by Louisa May Alcott, and one of her characters, Jo, changed my life. Jo, too, was snippy and snappish and determined to get a handle on her temper. Inspired by her hard work and ultimate success, I followed in her fictional footsteps. Of course I didn't realize it at the time, but Alcott via Jo was an excellent life-skills teacher!

The truth is that most people have no clue what life skills are or whether they possess them. It's not as if folks go to bed at night and ask themselves, "Gee, how'd I do with my life skills today?" Instead, they muddle through their days dodging difficulties, winging it, hoping for change and success, and fervently wishing that enlightenment and competence would suddenly descend on them. Moreover, too many folks display their skill deficiencies by tsk-tsking about the deficits of others rather than assessing and improving their own qualities.

As far as I can tell, the key factors in developing life skills are recognizing which ones you lack, being highly motivated to acquire them, and practice, practice, practice. (More on the importance of practice in a bit.) Of course, the earlier you jump on the life-skills bandwagon, the easier learning them will be. Our brains are most malleable in childhood, when they're being shaped or "pruned" by what we (often unconsciously) learn from other people and through the experiences we encounter. But the neural circuitry of our brains is far from fixed, and we can learn new tricks at any point in our lives.

How Does Motivation Affect My Ability to Learn Life Skills?

This is probably a good time to stop and consider how motivated you are to acquire the skills you're missing. Are you psyched, ambivalent, begrudgingly willing, or mildly enthusiastic; or do you feel as if you're dragging yourself through this book kicking and screaming? How will your drive level affect your ability to learn? What could you do to ratchet up your motivation? What do you suppose will happen if your enthusiasm remains low — or wanes?

Here are three steps to increase and sustain motivation:

Step 1. Recognize why you're not champing at the bit, ready to add new competencies to your repertoire, especially ones that not only will help you have a more positive relationship with food but also will undoubtedly enhance many areas of your life. Maybe you're scared that you won't succeed in learning them, that since you've already failed at reaching life goals so many times, you don't want to even bother trying. If so, let me assure you that as long as you have at least midlevel intelligence, there's nothing stopping you *but* a fear of failure — that is, there's no earthly reason why you won't be able to learn these skills over time. We're not talking quantum physics here but the everyday actions that you see being taken by intimates and strangers. So if you fear you won't succeed, lay that misconception to rest. Most important, push that fear out of your mind, because the one reason — the sole reason — you might fail is the belief that you will.

Step 2. Focus on what learning life skills will get you. Break down the rewards, rather than saying, "I'll eat better" or "I'll be happier." What do those words really mean in concrete terms? Write down ten specific changes that will happen when you have improved your life skills, such as: "I will choose more appropriate friends; I won't turn to food so much when I'm stressed; I'll be better able to handle distressing emotions; I'll make wiser decisions; I'll treat myself better; I won't feel so bored and dissatisfied with life." See what I mean? Get down to specifics so you can keep in mind the rewards you'll reap by sticking with the learning process.

Step 3. Stop thinking you have to learn all your skills perfectly — and right this minute. Instead, plan on letting the process inch along slowly but steadily. Helpful mantras include: "Baby steps, nothing but baby steps" and (my favorite) "I'm doing the best I can and that's all I can do." Perfection and impatience are the enemies of progress. They're the attitudes that will most likely make you think you can't learn and, therefore, cause you to stop trying. Expect learning to be frustrating, slow, and incremental, and you won't be disappointed. Cultivate realistic optimism that says your competence and expertise will come in good time — not in a short time.

Think of yourself as entering college or a training program. In your first semester, everything will be a bit new and mind-boggling and you'll feel at sea, thinking you'll never catch on to what you're supposed to learn. That's what the first semester is all about — learning how to learn — in terms of setting expectations and knowing how to pace yourself. You wouldn't expect to know, as a freshman, all that seniors know, would you? Okay, then, acknowledge that you're at the *beginning* of learning, not at the *end*, and don't fault yourself for not getting things right away. You're not supposed to, nor is anyone else. Learning is a process, not an event!

▰▰ Get Smart!

Do you believe you must know everything right away, and that if you don't you're a failure? Do you fear that everyone else will "get it" but you won't? How do these faulty beliefs affect your ability to learn and sustain your motivation? What beliefs could you develop to ensure that your thinking about learning is helpful and won't impede your progress?

How Do I Know What Life Skills I Need to Learn?

There are two answers to this question. The first, broad answer is that you have to learn *all* the life skills necessary to achieve your goals. The narrower answer is that you have to learn all the ones you lack. If you're like most folks, you probably do better in some areas than others. That said, life skills aren't optional, nor can you pick and choose among them as if they're items on a menu. It makes sense that the more skills you possess and the more proficient you are at using them, the better your life — and (not incidentally) your eating — will be. I've never met anyone with a solid set of life skills who continued to hang on to their eating difficulties. Having effective life skills makes *all* the difference.

The second and unique answer to the question of what you need to learn comes from your responses on the preassessment questionnaire. Based on the assumption that everyone needs all the itemized skills, you can identify the work you have ahead by noting the areas in which you could use improvement. Remember, there's no shame in admitting that you don't excel in every area — or in any area. If you did, you'd be doing something other than reading this book right now, wouldn't you? No one gets straight As when it comes to life skills, me included, I assure you. There's always something for us to learn and improve on. So, join the club!

How Long Will I Need to Practice before I Feel Adept at Life Skills?

This question assumes that all adults begin their learning on a level playing field. Nothing could be further from the truth. As I said previously, some fortunate folks have an excellent life-skills education growing up (acquired through family, relatives, school, community, and mentors) and some unfortunate folks are raised in environments that model and provide abysmal skills. So the answer to how long you need to practice must take your starting point into account.

In addition to assessing your current skill level by means of the preassessment questionnaire to determine how your progress might go, you'll want to answer these questions:

- Is my motivation strong enough to power me through the tough times of gradual skill learning?

- Do I already have abilities that can transfer from one life-skill area to another? (For example, if you're good at problem solving, acquiring other competencies may happen faster.)
- Am I able to ask for support and feedback as I learn these skills, or do I believe I must bumble along alone?
- If I'm not learning fast enough to meet my unrealistic expectations, will I call myself a failure and give up, or decide to plug along until I get it?
- Will my friends, family, or coworkers be supportive of my skill-learning process, or will they intentionally or unintentionally stand in the way?

Whatever your answers, I can assure you that life-skill learning will take longer than you hope it will. What learning doesn't? But so what? Since the time will fly by anyway, you might as well be doing something constructive to improve your relationship with food and then some. Even if you master only some of the skills, you'll be ahead of the game. Even if you remain at an intermediate skill level, you'll still be better off than you were as a novice. Don't talk yourself out of being able to succeed; instead, talk yourself into it!

If you really want to know how long it takes to gain proficiency in a subject, listen to what Malcolm Gladwell has to say in his enlightening book *Outliers: The Story of Success.* In it, he cites a study by psychologist Anders Ericsson, who carefully reviewed the histories of successful violinists at the Berlin Academy of Music and concluded that those who performed the best (according to judges) spent the most time practicing. Gladwell expands on this theory by asserting that ten thousand hours is the average number of hours the violinists spent practicing their craft in order to learn it. Ten thousand hours — equivalent to practicing straight through for almost 417 days, just shy of a year and two months' worth of solid practice time! He found this to be true, across the board, among other professionals learning their craft — athletes, composers, writers, artists, and even criminals.

Ericsson's and Gladwell's point is that *the one attribute that can catapult you to success in any discipline is the amount of practice time you are willing to put into it.* That practice makes progress is a highly hopeful assertion, because it helps cancel out the unevenness of the playing field we started on. In fact, practice is good news of the tallest order when it comes to learning life skills, proving that if you're hell-bent on learning how to build and maintain relationships, and refuse to give up before you've become an ace self-regulator or critical thinker, you will succeed. Taking this concept one step further, we might say that you can't help but succeed if you continue to practice, because the behaviors we do repeatedly — good, bad, or indifferent — are the ones that become habits. And the more we do 'em, the better we do 'em.

▰▰ Get Smart!

Assess your ability to remain motivated. When you slack off instead of practicing new learning, do you let yourself off the hook or, conversely, beat up on yourself? What excuses do you use when you don't want to practice? What rejoinder could you come up with to gently counter your excuses? (Remember, no "shoulds," puh-lease.)

Although there's been some research — based on the importance of certain genetic traits in learning and success — that challenges the ten-thousand-hour proficiency theory, I'd keep it in mind when you get tired of working hard to acquire a life skill, become frustrated that it's not coming easily, and want to throw in the towel and do things the old, more familiar way. If you wish to acquire new skills, whether eating or otherwise, you must keep practicing them. No matter what your history of dysfunction or trauma, if you are willing to keep on keeping on, mastery will be yours. You may be lucky — maybe proficiency will take you only nine thousand hours!

How Does Possessing or Lacking Life Skills Affect Eating, and Vice Versa?

How does it *not*? If you take a look at the life skills covered in this book, you'll see what I mean.

1. Skills for Wellness and Physical Self-Care

That's an easy one. If you don't have the concern and motivation necessary to take care of your body and keep it in excellent working order, eating unhealthily on a steady basis, or regularly overeating, isn't going to change. If you can't drag yourself off to bed when you're tired, or early enough to get a solid seven to nine hours' sleep most nights, you're more likely to have the munchies the next day, scientific studies say. If you tell yourself that you're hungry but too busy to eat breakfast, or if you usually skip lunch, you'll wind up so famished by dinner that you won't be able to prevent yourself from making poor food choices.

On the other hand, if you go to the doctor when you're sick or injured, you might head off physical problems that prevent you from being active (and you know what you'll end up doing if you're stuck in the house all day or night with nothing to do!). If you pay attention to physical messages from your body, you won't be as likely to stuff yourself with food when your body really wants rest and relaxation or to be charged up by activity. If you pride yourself in the terrific care you take of your body and your health, you won't think of engaging in abusing that well-valued body with food.

2. Skills for Handling Emotions

Need I say a great deal about the necessity of having skills to handle your emotions effectively? You know well enough what happens when you feel stressed or distressed, run from emotional discomfort, are sucked back into recalling old wounds, or are keyed up about your future — and feel confused and know no road to take but the one that passes by the cupboard with the Ring Dings. Having top-notch life skills for self-soothing — containing your feelings when appropriate, distracting yourself when necessary, pacing activities and demands so you don't get overly taxed, and comfortably asking for and accepting emotional support from others — goes a long way toward helping you become and remain a "normal" eater.

When you're emotionally challenged, life can devolve into a depressing quagmire, a minefield of crises that barely let you recover from one catastrophe before you're faced with the next. When you're emotionally skilled, you learn to avoid creating crises and know you can manage and bounce back from the few that come your way.

3. Skills for Living Consciously

Living on autopilot, not only do you make unwise choices, but you also generally dig yourself into the kind of deep holes from which it is difficult to climb out. You eat mindlessly, freak out, then starve yourself until you're almost too weak to pry off the top of a peanut butter jar. You say yes to requests you mean to decline, break plans at the last minute owing to exhaustion, and pinball from one day to the next without finding meaning in life or getting much enjoyment out of it. When you fail to take charge of your life, you end up feeling like a victim and treating yourself like one.

However, when you live out each moment with intention and attention, you're more engaged with the world. You don't miss danger signals warning that your relationships are not what you deserve, red flags that others can spot a mile away. Nor do you sleepwalk through life waiting and longing for some future event to rock your world. When you live consciously, you don't blame others for your poor choices, but take responsibility for growing and learning how to live up to your potential and strive to make each day better than the previous one.

As for food, when you live consciously, you eat only when you're hungry, and you recognize how to meet other needs effectively. You choose foods by considering their gustatory appeal and nutritional value. When you eat, you are mindful of every bite: you recognize how food tastes and feels in your body, realize when you are no longer hungry, and sense when you reach satisfaction. Mindful eating is an automatic outgrowth of conscious living.

4. Skills for Building and Maintaining Relationships

If we weren't meant to be interdependent, there wouldn't be so darned many of us on the planet. One of the key skill sets required for improving your relationship with food is improving your relationship with people. When you have the wherewithal to discern which folks are good relationship material for friends, dates, or mates; when you possess the know-how to both listen actively and share deeply and intimately; when you can hold others accountable yet not take everything personally; when you can tell others what you expect from them and live up to what they reasonably expect of you, then food will seem like a poor substitute for heart-to-heart human bonding.

Without these skills, you can't help but be disappointed, lonely, emotionally isolated, and more likely to make poor decisions, succumb to depression, and miss out on a great deal of fun. What you're more likely to do when you're sick at heart is to turn to food and perpetuate a vicious cycle that you know all too well. When you have only tenuous relational skills, food takes center stage while real life — the good life, your best life — is taking place somewhere off in the wings.

5. Skills for Self-Regulation

Whether you know it or not, if you are a compulsive and emotional binge eater, undereater, overeater, or chronic dieter, you lack adequate self-regulation skills. This means you have difficulty making small, incremental shifts in one direction or another to stay centered, to remain in balance, and to pace yourself well. I've never met a troubled eater who didn't have self-regulation difficulties regarding food and otherwise. A foolproof sign that you're not up to snuff with self-regulation is thinking and acting in all-or-nothing, extreme ways, or yo-yoing between the two, whether the subject is work, self-care, exercise, money, chores, fun, risk taking, commitment, drugs or alcohol, romance, or — you name it.

Self-regulation is a must-have skill for troubled eaters to develop. When you can sense what your mind or body is telling you and tune into "enoughness" (sufficiency), you'll be in better balance. You won't overdo, then underdo, and continue this yo-yo cycle. You won't fear excess or scarcity, too much freedom or too much structure. You'll feel more at peace and in sync with yourself and won't get exhausted ping-ponging back and forth between extremes. Plus, when you improve your skill at regulating yourself in nonfood areas, your proficiency can't help but rub off on your eating habits.

6. Skills for Problem Solving and Critical Thinking

You understand what the term *problem solving* means, but it's highly likely that you aren't sure what would be involved in acts of critical thinking. According to Dr. Ronald J. Massey, "These are sophisticated methods of assessing beliefs, opinions, and assertions using science, logic, and reliable information. Instead of simply accepting arguments and conclusions, one questions and evaluates in an organized manner."

Critical thinking teaches you how to separate fact from fiction, how to distinguish opinions from evidence-based truth, and how to put events and actions in context. A rigorous way of processing information that tells you the proof is in the pudding, critical thinking is pretty much the opposite of intuition and gut feeling. Too many people make important — more than that, critical — decisions based solely on how they *feel*. They screen out information that makes them uneasy using what's called confirmation bias — taking in only information that supports what they already believe or think — so that they need not be uncomfortable. They vote, pick jobs or partners, change jobs or partners, have children, parent, and plan entire lives without using rationality. Needless to say, mindless eating, or eating because you simply *feel* like it, is the antithesis of critical thinking.

When you start developing and utilizing critical-thinking skills, you'll begin making better decisions in all aspects of life. You'll weigh pros and cons, inform yourself of all your options and all their consequences, seek out evidence even if it makes you uncomfortable or shows you are wrong, recognize what's best for you rather than what feels good in the moment, and be willing to change your mind when facts point you in a different or better direction. Can you imagine living so skillfully and rationally? More important, can you imagine eating so skillfully and rationally?

7. Skills for Setting and Reaching Goals

The skills for setting and reaching goals encompass more than simply saying you want to do something, then charging off to do it. How many times have you gotten yourself up to the starting gate of "normal" eating and begun moving forward, only to falter before you've made it halfway through your first course? How often have you vowed to eat this and not eat that, and had the idea fly out of your head at the initial taste of this or that?

Without effective goal-setting skills and a clear understanding of the science and art of sustaining motivation and making progress, you're doomed to fail. And, if you're reading this book, you've had enough failures with food and weight goals to last ten lifetimes. Learning how to establish doable goals, divide big ones into smaller ones, reenergize yourself when your spirits flag, pace yourself, and recover from disappointment will go a long way toward helping you establish a positive relationship with food.

8. Skills for Balancing Work and Play

You might not have thought so, but balancing work and play demands skill, and a lack of competence in this area often triggers unwanted eating. Too much work and skyrocketing stress can send you straight to the cookie jar. Too much play and you may lose your ability to mobilize your inner resources and forget that life (and eating) have consequences. Moreover, one significant problem of dysregulated eaters is that eating is their major sport and passion — that is, it's how they break loose and let it all hang out. In fact, most troubled eaters are pretty much at square one when it comes to letting their hair down in effective, appropriate ways.

When you *intentionally* make a choice to work or play, you don't end up playing when you really wish to be working, or procrastinating so much that when it's time to play you need to hunker down and get work done pronto. As you can see, balancing work and play uses self-regulation skills and skills from living consciously. The more skilled you become at sensing what you need in terms of goal-directed activity (what we call work) and mindless fun (what we call play), the less you will turn to food to provide you with whichever you're lacking.

▰▰ Get Smart!

Using my list of life skills, rank them in order of your proficiency with each, starting with the category you do best with and ending with the category that needs your attention the most.

I hope I've convinced you that by learning and perfecting eight essential skills, you'll forever change your eating habits and your life. Every time you turn to people rather than food for comfort; give your body the exquisite care it deserves; make a well-informed, rational decision; create balance in your life; plug away at reaching a worthwhile goal; and keep yourself centered and grounded no matter what craziness is going on around you, you grow wiser. And each hard-earned bit of wisdom will make skill-building that much easier and bring you closer to outsmarting overeating.

Skill Boosters

1. Read over the eight categories of life skills every day and work toward identifying when you are doing one or another. You might think, "Ah, critical-thinking skills are what I need right now," "Gee, I see some red flags in this relationship," or "I'm doing pretty well at self-regulating today."

2. Pick out one or two (three at most) skills to work on — say, problem solving and physical self-care, or building relationships and balancing work and play — and focus on developing them for one week. Then pick other skill sets for another week.

3. Notice the life skills of other people and consider whether they're better or worse than you'd expect. Pay special attention to people with excellent life skills and emulate them.

4. Make a list of the life skills you need or wish to improve in order to eat more "normally." If you engage in unwanted eating, recognize which skills you're not employing effectively enough — say, self-soothing when you're upset, playing enough, or asking others for help with your problems. Then put special attention on using these skills to improve your eating.

5. Make a list of skills you excel at — say, sociability, working effectively, creativity, parenting, athletic prowess — and read them over every day. Be detailed and specific when citing your skills — not "I'm good with people" but "I'm an

attentive listener; not "I'm a pretty fair tennis player" but "I have a wicked backhand." These examples will help you feel less inadequate as you learn the skills in this book, by reminding you of how many things you already do well.

6. Monitor your motivation, and remember that it takes some ten thousand hours to become highly proficient at a skill. Notice when your motivation revs up and when it wanes, and reflect on what triggers the shift. Do more of what keeps you motivated and less of what doesn't. When you get impatient, focus on the present and what you've already achieved. Make sure to note all progress, tiny as it may seem, rather than focusing exclusively, as most dysregulated eaters do, on what you have yet to accomplish.

In chapter 2, you'll learn how to take care of your body from head to toe to improve your quality of life and longevity.

CHAPTER 2

Wellness and Physical Self-Care

You Mean My Body's Not Like a Self-Cleaning Oven?

Taking care of your body is the life skill closest to eating healthfully. You might not even consider this a skill and instead may just take it for granted that, like an oven, your body will take care of itself. It may seem to, if you're in the bloom of youth — say, in your late teens or early twenties, when humans are in peak condition, their physical prime. But to get beyond that point and maintain some semblance of wellness for the rest of your days takes a substantial amount of consistent care.

That care starts in the womb, where, if you were fortunate, you didn't have toxic substances like alcohol, harmful drugs, and unhealthy foods dumped into your fetal bloodstream. And you weren't subjected to high amounts of cortisol from Mother's frequent and intense bouts of anxiety, fear, or anger. Instead, you were lovingly and safely ensconced inside her until you were ready to make your grand entrance into the world.

If your stars continued to align, you grew from an infant into a youth whose physical needs were taken seriously. If you had a boo-boo and it warranted a bandage (sometimes even if it didn't), you got one. Your parents and other relatives put great attention on preventing accidents from happening to you and took pains to grow you strong and healthy. They lathered you in sunscreen so that you wouldn't burn and harmful UV rays wouldn't damage your sensitive skin. They bundled you up from head to toe before you went out in the cold and snow and cozied you under their umbrella when it rained.

They took you to the doctor or dentist for regular checkups and to the hospital in emergencies. You received appropriate vaccinations, were compelled to take your medicine no matter how much you screamed and yelled (or hid from it), and were taught how to more or less stay out of harm's way. For example, your parents may have allowed you to climb trees but go only so far up, to play on your swing set but soar only so high, and to ride a bike or roller-skate but nowhere near heavily trafficked roads. As I tick off this list, you may take these things for granted, whereas others would start to notice that their parents, in fact, didn't make many of these necessary efforts.

There's another kind of physical care that speaks volumes about how much your caretakers valued you, their child: making sure that you sat in a car seat until you no longer *legally* needed one, seeing that you buckled up your seat belt every time you got into the car, and ensuring that you wore a helmet when you were bike riding, roller-skating, or skiing. Actions like these speak volumes about how your parents valued you. They say, "You are so precious to me, so vital to my happiness and well-being, that I will do whatever is in my power to keep you safe." The message that would have come across to you, the young child, is this: I am loved, precious, of great significance and value to someone else; therefore, I must be lovable, precious, and valuable.

If parents are smokers it's unhealthy for them to smoke around their child, because the message this conveys is: "My pleasure and comfort are more important than your health." If parents must smoke, they should do it outdoors or at least not in rooms their children generally occupy. Having a parent step outside to have a cigarette says to a child, "Right now I can't help mistreating *my* body, but I'm sure as heck not going to mistreat *yours*." (We'll get to confusing double messages regarding parental care versus child care in just a moment.)

One thing parents should never do is to hit or strike a child in any way. This reaction causes all kinds of problems, the obvious ones being that, if your parents struck you, they were not in control of themselves and were not taking the time to communicate with you effectively. Another obvious problem with hitting children is that it hurts and can damage them, and if done repeatedly it can dysregulate a child's nervous system. A slap on the head, a jab in the chest, a punch in the stomach — any of these actions can do real, though unintended, harm. Moreover, your parents crossed a line if they mistreated your body, because it gave you a double message. Maybe they slapped you because you frightened them when you ran into traffic, but the slap is confusing because it says, "I'm hurting you so you don't hurt yourself." Huh? A perplexing message at best and one that children internalize as: "It's okay to hurt my body if it's done in the service of taking care of it." It doesn't take a genius to see how that kind of mentality can lead to eating problems down the road — for example, to thinking that starving yourself is okay because it leads to a low weight, which is supposed to be healthy.

One more instance of how your parents may have unintentionally taught you that your body has little worth was by being neglectful. Maybe they were busy working two or three jobs or caring for your siblings or their elderly parents. Maybe they had their own physical or mental disabilities to deal with and they did what they could, but it was the bare minimum. Neglectful parents may have forgotten your doctor or dental appointments, pooh-poohed taking you to the emergency room even when you were badly injured (especially if it would have inconvenienced them), didn't make you take your medicine, or didn't refill your prescriptions on time. I'm not saying that parents intentionally fail to take physical care of their children; but whatever the reason, the impact is often the same. As a child, what you intuited from their actions (or, in this case, their lack of action) was that your body and well-being didn't matter awfully much so you must not be worth very much to them. ·

You may think I'm making too big a fuss over the specifics of how your parents took care of you physically and kept you well. What I mean to convey is less the significance of each specific act and more the aggregate impact: what is communicated by these actions during your first two decades of life. If you weren't made to wear a helmet while roller-skating, it doesn't mean your parents didn't love you or didn't care if you injured your body. Ditto if they didn't always reslather you with sunscreen after you finished swimming and toweled off. However, I cannot stress strongly enough that, aside from its importance to your health, *how your parents cared for your body went a long way toward teaching you how to value it.* If they neglected or mistreated your body, there is a good chance that you will too! Enough said on that subject.

■■■ Get Smart!

How well did your parents take care of your body, not just your health; how well did they protect you from physical harm? Were they attentive or neglectful? What lessons did you learn from how they treated your minor or major health concerns? How do those lessons play out in your care of your health and body today?

What If Parents Take Care of Their Children's Bodies but Don't Take Care of Their Own?

If your parents took care of your body, but not theirs, they gave you a perplexing message: "Do as I say, not as I do." Children not only pick up information from how they're treated, but they also infer what to think and do from what they observe. For example, I knew a woman who would always carefully strap her toddler into her car with a seat belt but would never wear one herself. One day, I was driving her child somewhere alone when she blurted out, "How come Mommy makes me wear a seat belt but she never does?" How come indeed? Think about how confusing this is for a young child to sort out: the most important person in her life (her parent), whose behavior the child unconsciously watches like a hawk, fails to take care of her own body but makes sure to take the utmost care of her child's body.

How would a child interpret this contradictory behavior? She'd wonder why her body is so important but her mother's is less so. Does this mean that children are more important and should be better treated than grown-ups? Does it mean that when she becomes an adult she has to take care of her child's body, but she can slack off when it comes to her own? Should she do as her beloved parents do, in order to be like them, or should she do what is done to her by them? My head is spinning just writing about such puzzling dilemmas.

The message is also wildly confusing when parents lavish care on their own bodies but not on those of their children. They rush off to the doctor or take medication for every minor ache and pain, but ignore their children's fevers and even broken bones. What a terrible message that gives to a child: I, your parent, am worthy and valuable, and you, my child, are not.

A child needs to receive congruent messages from her parents: they take good physical care of her and of themselves. If she is to value her body, however, the message must be positive. Too often parents neglect their own bodies and health and those of their children. This is a heart-breaker of a message, but at least it's clear: bodies have little value, so why bother to care for them?

▰▰ Get Smart!

Were there any double messages about wellness and physical self-care when you were growing up? What messages did you receive? How do the messages you received affect your physical self-care today? What impact have they had on your eating or weight?

What If I Don't Like Going to the Doctor or the Dentist?

Please don't be offended, but this kind of question comes from not using critical-thinking skills. In fact, it's a great example of how people don't employ these skills to take care of their health. Over the decades I've heard this question countless times, more than I can recall, in fact. The question suggests that there are people who actually go wild over being poked and prodded with stethoscopes and needles by a relative stranger while sitting stiffly and devoid of clothing on a paper-covered sterile table in an office the temperature of an igloo. It also suggests that some strange folks positively swoon over flu shots and stress tests, never mind biopsies and colonoscopies.

Okay, you get my drift. Whether you like going to the doctor or the dentist is so beside the point. The point is that you go because you care about your physical well-being and are determined to stay as healthy as possible for as long as possible. Truly, I'm the first person to say that feelings have their place in life. But using them to make health care decisions is not one of them. You can't live your best life when you're guided by fear and discomfort. Getting medical or dental attention has nothing to do with how you feel about the *activity*, and everything to do with how you feel about *yourself*!

What If My Health and Body Are Such a Mess That I'm Clueless about How to Start Taking Care of Myself?

I run into many clients who have let their health go so far that the thought of taking stock of their myriad ailments and learning how to properly deal with them makes them just want to cry. I sympathize, but that's not what these folks need. Nor do you. The best I can offer is hope and encouragement that, by taking small steps, you will feel a lot better both physically and emotionally. One problem is that you may not know where to begin — which doctor to call first, how to find a competent dentist who doesn't charge an arm and a leg, what annual tests to have for your age and gender, and how much insurance will pay for and what comes out of pocket. And another problem is that you may feel you have to make every appointment tomorrow or the next day, and you're afraid that if you don't you're going to put things off and these medical visits will never happen.

I recommend a few starting strategies. First, find a primary care doctor you like — really like — not just someone your neighbor raves about or the first name in the phone book or on your insurance plan. You have the right to doctor shop for high-quality medical care. Doctor or hospital shopping can be time-consuming, of course, but it's not impossible. Although you can't meet every physician and dentist available, you can go online and check out whatever information you can find on them, especially of the lawsuit and patient satisfaction variety. I know that sounds hypervigilant, but it's a place to start. Also, some communities — like mine — put out booklets that rate health practitioners. Try asking everyone you know for a referral that includes why they specifically like the health care professional they're recommending, as well as anything they don't care for about him or her.

Think about what's important to you: the doctor's expertise or specialization, gender, good listening skills, bedside manner, office hours, and proximity to your home; the ease of getting an appointment; the length of a visit; cost; after-hours availability or back-up coverage; how well the office is managed; and so on. If possible, be picky. I went to two primary care doctors after I moved from Boston to Sarasota, before finding a third one, with whom I was happy. Unless you live in a rural area with few health care providers, the more you know about what you want from one, the better you'll do at finding the right person. By the way, I suggest that, unless you're in an emergency situation, you start with identifying a primary care doctor before any others. Usually he or she can recommend specialists.

If you haven't been to the doctor in a long time, you might be fretting about what he or she will say about such a lapse, and this may incline you toward putting off making an appointment. If this is the case, you're proving my point about a need for improved life skills. For example, if you were better at self-soothing, you wouldn't be so anxious about a relatively innocuous, routine medical visit. If you were using effective problem-solving or critical-thinking skills, you wouldn't be struggling while deciding whether to avoid emotional discomfort by not going to the doctor or to ignore your anxiety and get your butt there posthaste. If you were living in the moment and not in the past or future, you wouldn't be ruminating about all the things the last doctor said to do that you didn't get done, or agitating about what your new doctor will think of your weight or poor health.

Your best bet is to make one or two appointments at a time — no more — so you don't get overwhelmed. Start with generalists. Take notes or, as soon as you leave the office, make a summary of what's been said. Better yet, see if you can get someone to go with you to jot down important points. Heads up: schedule your next appointment before you leave the office. This is where many folks fall down on the job. They forget their appointment book or digital device and say they'll call when they get home and don't. Repeat: do not leave the medical office without having scheduled your next visit. Better to reschedule it at a later date if it proves inconvenient than not to have an appointment at all.

If you don't know what kinds of tests you need, given your age and gender, ask the doctor. Or go online and see what's recommended by reputable sites. Try to schedule required tests as soon as possible (so you don't build up anxiety waiting for them). Write the test dates on a calendar, not on a scrap of paper that you might mistake for an old receipt and toss out. And if you don't schedule your next appointment ahead of time, then on your calendar, on the month before the appointment needs to take place, make a note to remind yourself to schedule it. For example, if you have your teeth cleaned every three months, and you last went in April, jot a note to yourself on the June page of your calendar about scheduling your next cleaning for July.

This is not rocket science here. It's using management and planning skills to take care of something you value — your health and body. You might think I'm crazy for being so picayune about all this health care minutiae, but many dysregulated eaters are so used to not taking care of their medical concerns that they lack the organizational skills to do so.

I suspect that you may have concerns that relate to your size, shape, and weight that keep you from getting medical attention. However, there are plenty of "normal" weight folks who take inadequate care of their bodies, and under- and overweight people who practice excellent physical self-care. Moreover, devaluing your body most likely preceded your eating problems and is the real issue: that is, thinking too little of yourself to carefully monitor and manage your health.

And while you're doctor shopping, it's important to think about obtaining health insurance coverage. In a practical sense, you will likely need it in the long run. Moreover, it says that you value yourself enough to spend money on making sure you can pay to have your medical concerns taken care of. And it speaks volumes about your ability to problem solve and use critical-thinking skills. The time to think of unexpected occurrences is not while they're happening but before they happen.

What about Everyday Stuff That Shows I Care about My Physical Self?

I wish I had a dollar for every client I've heard complain about how much trouble it is to take care of himself or herself physically. Is that how you feel? Here are activities that appear to be the most burdensome: doing laundry, food shopping, cooking, keeping living quarters clean and neat, getting enough sleep, following a skin care regimen, practicing dental hygiene, taking vitamins, and buying and wearing appropriate size, comfortable clothes and shoes.

Wearing well-fitting clothes and shoes is a must, because it keeps your focus off what you're not wild about regarding your body — its size. Dressing suitably and attractively is part of daily physical self-care as well. I don't mean that you have to get all dolled or suited up to run across the street to grab a quart of milk in the 7-Eleven. I do mean making sure your clothes are clean and they fit well. Your shoes too. I understand that large people often have difficulty finding comfy footgear, but these days you can shop online for them and, at some sites, even get free shipping. Shoes are important: they ferry your body around all day long.

Clean, pressed clothes speak volumes about who you think you are. There's a huge difference between someone who's dressed attractively and well-kept and one who isn't — at any weight. Next time you go out, pay attention to well-appointed people and notice how you feel about them at first sight. Forget their size or shape; just notice their general appearance and the message it sends out. Telling yourself you're too fat or thin to dress nicely fools no one but yourself and is called pretzel logic. C'mon, does that really compute? If you're unhappy with your body, why compound your perceived problem by not looking presentable?

Getting Your Zzs

Most of us need between seven and nine hours' sleep most nights to function well. If you get less, your hormones will go awry, specifically the ones that influence your appetite. Sleep deficiency causes increased production of ghrelin, which generates sensations of hunger, and decreased production of leptin, which promotes satiation. If that isn't exactly the opposite of what you, as an overeater, want to happen, I don't know what is. I hate to push, but if there's one positive self-care action to take for your body, it's getting enough sleep.

Caring for Your Teeth, Skin, and Hair

When you're in a rush in the morning or exhausted at night, it can feel like a drag to pay attention to your teeth and gums, which means any or all of the following: brushing, flossing, rinsing, irrigating. If you don't continue to bemoan how long and boring the process is, you could probably do the whole shebang in about five minutes, give or take. That's ten minutes every day, and all of us can carve out that itty-bitty amount of time for oral hygiene. I bet you spend more time than that reading emails, posting on Facebook, and texting your friends. Need I say more?

I'm going to throw skin and hair care into the it's-too-much-trouble-so-I-don't-bother-with-it category. Again, we're talking about minutes at a time. Washing your face in the morning and evening (preferably with a clean washcloth, because dermatologists tell us that wet washcloths carry gross bacteria), using sunscreen before you go out and reapplying it during the day, and finding a moisturizer that will keep your skin feeling and looking fresh are all important. You don't need to spend hours fussing and primping, nor your entire paycheck on high-end products. Just the basics will take you a long way.

As to hair care, ask a stylist how often you need to wash your particular type of hair. Lose the all-or-nothing mentality, as in: No one's looking at my hair because they're staring at my ugly body, so why should I bother? A better perspective is to feel good about your haircut or hairstyle and not obsess so much about your body. Work on directing people's attention to what *you* want them to see about your appearance. Here's a case in point: I was at a local blues club not long ago when a singer stepped onto the stage. She probably weighed well over three hundred pounds, and she had long, well-styled, shiny black hair and a modest amount of makeup, which emphasized her startling green eyes. The sparkly red top she was wearing was a knockout. And as soon as she belted out her first number, I can tell you, the audience was all ears.

One more point about appearance and I'll move on. I'm not saying that females must wear makeup. That's a personal choice and, for some, even a feminist issue. No woman has to wear eyeliner, blush, or lipstick to be attractive, and those who overdo may be expressing fear that they're not good-looking enough to go out in public without a little of this and a lot of that. Do whatever makes you feel attractive.

Creating a Peaceful Living Space

What, you might be wondering, does maintaining a peaceful living space have to do with physical self-care? I know if you think a minute, you'll come up with the answer. If your surroundings are pleasant to look at, you have a better shot at wanting to make the person who's living in them pleasant to look at as well. Sometimes when I meet someone who's poorly groomed, I come to find out that his or her house or apartment (or dorm room) is, quite frankly, a mess. Again, it's all about what you value. On the other hand, I've often been surprised to find that someone who seems as if he or she has not looked in a mirror in a long, long while lives in an environment that is lovely, attractive, neat, and creative. That tells me something too: this person loves beauty but doesn't feel that his or her body deserves it. Sadly, this person has an eye for attractiveness and good taste that gets turned outward, toward decor, and not inward, toward his or her body.

Buying and Making Food

I left grocery shopping, meal planning, and food preparation to the end of this section intentionally, because many dysregulated eaters feel a crushing fatigue and go mentally offline at the mere mention of what they call these "chores." What is it about the natural task of feeding your body that seems so grueling? Why do you have such antipathy toward activities that are so routine for most people? That is, many folks may not adore shopping and cooking, but they do it because they enjoy eating and know they're responsible for feeding themselves.

The problem is that some people feel they don't deserve to eat well, and so they deny their bodies pleasurable nourishment. Others wish someone would swoop in and make their meals for them so they'd feel well taken care of. Still others get so overwhelmed thinking about what's "right" to buy or cook that they give up before they're out the door and end up noshing on whatever's in the kitchen.

■■■ Get Smart!

How would you rate your daily physical self-care? What activities are you proud of doing well and consistently? Which ones could you put more effort into? What gets in the way of taking excellent physical care of your body each and every day? What excuses do you use? How will you change your thinking to make these activities more appealing and integral to your life? Do you tell yourself the problem is your eating or weight or time or money, when it's really about how little you value yourself?

How Do I Develop Better Skills for Wellness and Physical Self-Care?

The first thing to do is to remind yourself that you've learned many skills throughout your lifetime, which means there are many things you do well, even exceptionally well. Very often the activities we're good at come easily to us, but sometimes not. I heard an interview with the late Lester Young, a saxophone great, on NPR not long ago in which he was complaining about how hard it was for him to learn to read music. It came naturally to his siblings, but not to him, though he could play by ear. However, reading music was a requirement if he wanted to play in the family band, so he painstakingly taught himself how to do it. Even at the time of the interview, he didn't much like doing it, but he understood the value of being a proficient music reader.

Learning to take better care of yourself physically cannot possibly be any harder than it was for Lester Young to become adept at reading music. The initial step comes from deciding how important this skill is to you. I will say that if you want to become a "normal" eater and be comfortable in and with your body, then becoming more skilled at physical self-care will be a gentle lead-in to it. If your dental and skin care are first-class, if you take pains with how you look because doing so is a reflection of how you feel about yourself, if you get a solid night's sleep most nights, and if you make sure that your environment is attractive, it will be a lot easier to ease into enhancing your feeding capabilities.

My point is that sometimes you have to set the stage for major change and let it come to you, rather than attack it head-on as if you're out to conquer the badlands. Start with making improvements in your physical arena (that means your body and the space you occupy a good part of the time), and it will feel more natural to care diligently for yourself. If you're stumped about how to dress up or spruce up your living quarters, ask a friend who has a flair for design and decor. Creative people generally love helping friends spiff up anything, anywhere. Don't be shy. You'll be doing some artistic person a favor; moreover, the more time you spend with this person, the more you'll see things through his or her eyes. You'll begin to notice what works and what doesn't, a skill in itself. Remember, people go to school to learn how to do this (although, to be fair, some folks seem to be born with the knack).

There are other practical ways to develop physical self-care skills. Make a folder for each of your health practitioners in which to file your appointment notes and test results; keep a calendar just for medical and dental visits or for regular appointments for haircuts and the like. Go through your closet at least twice a year to get rid of old clothes and bundle them up for the consignment store or to donate to charity. Have a clothes swap with friends or work colleagues at least annually. I once gave an adorable pair of loafers to a friend because they looked so wrong on my feet and so right on hers. I got a kick out of seeing her wear them.

Notice what other people are wearing, and make a mental note if you think you'd look good in that style or color. You don't have to spend a fortune on clothes, believe me. I confess that I'm a clotheshorse and buy over 50 percent of what's in my crammed closet at either consignment stores or Goodwill. I rarely pay full price for clothes.

So that you don't "forget" daily (or weekly) living activities, make a chart of everyday tasks and check them off: dental care, check; skin care, check; vitamins, check; laundry, check; dust, vacuum, mop, check. I have a client who has numerous health problems, but boy does she have a great system for taking her medication. She keeps all her pills in a box in the refrigerator, affixed to which is her pill-popping schedule and a pencil on a string. It can't get any simpler, or more doable, than that.

When it comes to food shopping and preparation, you might find yourself being squeamish or uneasy about stepping up to the plate (pun intended). That's because, as I mentioned earlier, feeding and nourishing yourself may be fraught with underlying conflict. Still, there are steps you can take. First and foremost, for goodness' sake, quit telling yourself how you hate to shop and cook. A former client spent every session telling me all about her abhorrence of anything related to grocery shopping and food preparation, then couldn't imagine why she avoided these opportunities for self-nurturing. Every word she uttered reinforced her negativity. Note: Tell yourself how you want to be tomorrow, not how you were yesterday or are today.

So, lighten up and brighten up. Find something pleasant about each task. In the supermarket, notice that you're getting exercise, enjoying a chance to people-watch, or just plain getting out of the house. As you're placing items in your cart, smile and tell yourself that what you're doing is part of taking care of yourself and those you love. Remind yourself that you're proud of going the extra mile to feed your body well. Keep smiling and staying positive — it's hard to feel resentful or angry when you're smiling. Vow never to tell yourself how much you can't stand these tasks. They're not odious; they're expressions of self-love.

As to cooking, I'm not a "foodie" and never will be. I confess that I keep it simple except when I have dinner guests, but I try to make mealtime or snacks tasty and nourishing. If you're unskilled in the feed-yourself department, get a 1-2-3 easy cookbook, take a class, or ask a friend who can cook to teach you how. Start out eating what you enjoy that's easy to make. Honestly, most of us eat the same things over and over anyway. Some people find this mostly satisfying (me, for instance), while others easily get bored. The way I see it, that's why there are restaurants (and doggy bags).

Someone asked me the other day what I think about when a large serving of food is placed in front of me in a restaurant. What else, but how many meals it might save me from making! Collect restaurant coupons and treat yourself once in a while, or occasionally get reasonably priced take-out; and if your appetite can manage it, make two meals out of one. Cook a bunch of stuff over the weekend and freeze it for the week ahead. Ask family members to take turns cooking or grocery shopping to give you a break.

Potluck with neighbors. Whatever you do in the food department, remind yourself that it's like sending a care package from you to you, one based on pure love and an uncrushable desire to be well and healthy.

So That's All There Is to It?

Well, no, not exactly. All the earlier suggestions will make it easier for you to become skillful at physical self-care, but they won't work if you're ambivalent about your self-worth. Sorry, but that's the way the cookie crumbles. If you harbor mixed feelings about your value as a human being and what you deserve, you may struggle with treating yourself well within, and outside of, the food arena. You may fail to act on any of the suggestions I've given here, or (more likely) you may do some of them for a while, then give up and go back to not attending to your physical needs. Then at some point, something will spur you to resume these routines, and, at another point, something else will cause you to drop them like a hot potato. You know how it is: you're in the groove until, poof, suddenly you're not. In no time flat, you go from self-care to "I don't care."

If you're curious about how you can get off this seesaw, that's the ticket. You're becoming skilled at problem solving, not merely sitting around lamenting what a sorry excuse for a human being you are. To end yo-yo behavior, you have to quit yo-yo thinking and, once and for all, come to a decision: Is you is or is you ain't, as the saying goes — worth it, that is. If you harbor doubts, you'll have to understand why, explore them, and toss them out with the garbage. Read self-help books, get into therapy, or join a support group. *You can't continue to be ambivalent about your value as a human being and expect to move forward and stay there.*

It's perfectly possible to go from conflicted to unconflicted. For years, I had self-worth conflicts, and now have none. I feel 100 percent worthy of the best in life 100 percent of the time. This change didn't happen overnight, but through an organic process. I went through it, and you can too. I assure you that when you're more single-minded about your value, self-care will be oodles easier. For more detailed instruction on how to use the organic process and resolve internal conflicts, read my book *Starting Monday: Seven Keys to a Permanent, Positive Relationship with Food.*

Beware: You can't sit around waiting to feel unconflicted, but must start acting this minute as if you know what you're doing is best for you. This means pretending or imagining and soon believing that you're just as deserving of health and happiness as anyone else on the planet. I suspect you'll say, "But how do I *know* it's true?" Clients ask me this question all the time. They don't know, and neither do you. But you don't know that you're a worthless sack of sand, either. You fake it 'til you make it, and if you're not willing to do that, I guarantee you won't make it. You live in a way that's called "as if " — as if you were everything you want to be or think you should be, as if you're the greatest thing since sliced bread, as if you're the king or queen of the universe. Then gradually that's what you become.

Get Smart!

What's your current motivation to learn skills for wellness and physical self-care? What do you tell yourself that moves you forward? What do you say that prevents you from moving forward? Which physical skills will be easy to pick up? Which ones will be a challenge? Who can you recruit to help you?

Skill Boosters

1. Reflect on the physical and health care you received as a newborn and as a child, and see if there's a connection between your treatment back then and how you treat your body now. If you weren't well taken care of physically, that means you never learned the skills you need, and you must stop blaming yourself for being a failure.

2. Consider the double messages you might have received about physical self-care, and begin to sort them out. These messages can be crazy-making if you try to straighten them out on your own, so, by all means, talk them out with someone you trust and let them help you. Then figure out how to retain only the message that is most constructive and beneficial for you.

3. Are there any health care appointments (medical, dental, tests) you need to make? Write them down, find the phone numbers you need, and put the list by the phone. Could you make one call right now? Rather than thinking of how anxious you are about making an appointment, think about how proud you'll feel after you do.

4. Pick one area of daily-living skills to take on — food shopping and preparation, keeping your living quarters clean and neat, getting enough sleep, caring for your skin and teeth, or dressing appropriately — and visualize how you will improve. Focus on the pride you'll feel after you've done your weekly grocery shopping or your laundry or cleaned the house.

5. If you're not sure you think well enough of yourself to treat yourself like the awesome person you are, figure out why before attempting to acquire new skills. It's fine to spend time doing this before jumping on the skills bandwagon. In fact, it's more than fine; it's necessary. Resolve your mixed feelings, and learning new skills will come far more easily. Therapy helps.

In chapter 3, you'll learn what it means to have effective emotional management by building inner resources and getting support.

CHAPTER 3

Handling Emotions

I Thought That's What a Spoon and Fork Were For!

You may never have thought that handling emotions effectively involves skill, and you may assume that some people are simply born better at it than you are. Maybe you've been amazed at how they seem to keep it together in the most depressing or hair-raising situations, or at how appropriately restrained they appear to be under one set of circumstances and assertive and dogged in another. Perhaps you envy the passionate, fully engaged lives that friends, family members, colleagues, or acquaintances enjoy without their becoming emotionally drained or overwhelmed. Maybe you're in awe of how people seemingly magically rebound from the most tragic events. I bet you never thought of their successes as skill based.

Yes, handling emotions effectively is a skill, or rather a set of skills that are learnable by anyone at any age. If you've experienced difficulty regulating emotions, I recommend that you read *The Food and Feelings Workbook: A Full Course Meal on Emotional Health*, which I wrote specifically for emotional eaters. I guarantee that it will vastly improve the way you manage stress and distress — and eating! But when I tell you there's a correlation between food and feelings, don't simply take my word for it. Here's what Robert E. Thayer, PhD, author of *Calm Energy: How People Regulate Mood with Food and Exercise*, has to say: "In my view, if you forget everything else — including the kinds of food to eat, their relative proportions and exact amounts — but you master your moods, you will go a long way toward controlling overeating."

What are these things we call emotions? Here's a scientific perspective. In her enlightening and delightful memoir, *My Stroke of Insight: A Brain Scientist's Personal Journey*, neuroanatomist Jill Bolte Taylor, PhD, writes about her amazing journey back from a massive stroke and talks a great deal about emotions along the way. The book is both deeply personal and unflinchingly scientific. Taylor maintains that it takes "less than 90 seconds" for an emotion to get triggered, surge chemically through the bloodstream, then get flushed out. "What, emotions are chemicals?" you're thinking. "And the chemicals get discharged in under a minute and a half? Who'd have thunk it!" She goes on to assert that within this brief period of time, the automatic emotional response generates and arrives at completion, so that *whatever we feel after that is of our choosing*. Now that's something to think about, isn't it?

Let's look at an example of this process, taken from something that happened to one of my clients, who gave me a blow-by-blow description of a workplace problem he'd encountered decades before. He had worked for a company in which serious ethical violations had been going on for some time. Unbeknownst to management, he and his coworkers had contacted the company's board of directors to advise them of the violations and asked that they root out the rotten apples involved. At one point in a staff meeting, the head honcho (the rottenest apple of all!) looked around the table, making sure to stop and glare at each and every employee while breathing fire — or so my client swore! The boss announced that he'd heard rumors that a few employees were unhappy, and that he wanted them to identify themselves then and there and speak their minds.

Here's how my client described feeling. *Boom*, his heart started pounding like a drum and his face felt as if it were on fire. He couldn't catch his breath, and his boss's voice sounded oddly muffled and far away. The feeling didn't last long; my client estimated that it went on for — you guessed it — about ninety seconds. After that, his heart rate began to slow down, his face cooled, and his breathing slowly returned to normal. Of course, he was still upset and feared being found out — and fired on the spot. Nothing of the kind happened. He reported no one noticing that he felt he might expire in his chair and never live to see the results of his office mutiny (which, by the way, was an empowering success).

For those of us who've held on to grief, grudges, ingratitude, rejection, insults, abandonment, bitterness, and the like for years or decades, Dr. Taylor's take on emotions may sound astonishing or even unbelievable. Even to someone like me who's spent decades in the field of psychology, the idea that an emotion from start to finish lasts for only about a minute and a half (far less time than it takes to do a respectable job of brushing my teeth with my electric toothbrush!) is astounding news with mind-blowing implications. It means that emotions function on a physical level that can be measured and monitored and are not all "in our heads." They're nothing but chemical surges that course through us like electrical currents. In fact, when you think about it, that's often how an emotion feels: a flash of searing pain, followed by rapidly escalating distress that floods through us and then, suddenly, recedes, similar to the reaction you get from an injection at the doctor's office. You wince an "ouch!" when the needle pierces your skin, and the pain surges, peaks, then dissipates. In no time flat, the ordeal is over.

What's the Best Way to React to Emotions?

The first thing to do when you have a feeling is to notice it — really notice it — and see if you can give it a name. Noticing means *acknowledging* that something is going on inside you. Don't pretend that nothing's wrong. Just let it happen. Remember, the chemical reaction of the emotion will be over within ninety seconds. Don't try to push away the feeling (a.k.a. avoidance), pretend it's no big deal (a.k.a. minimizing), explain it away (a.k.a. rationalizing), or switch to thinking mode rather than feeling mode (a.k.a. intellectualizing). Simply experience whatever is occurring within you, without having a gazillion judgments about it, especially about whether you should, or want to, be having the emotion or not. Think of it this way: If someone stomps on your foot, you feel pain, pure and simple. You don't spend time considering if you're better off not feeling the pain or what kind of ninny you are to have such a sensitive foot.

Dr. Taylor encourages us to be scientists like her, curious and totally nonjudgmental about what we're feeling. After all, emotions, like our senses, are meant only to guide us in the world. They're similar to musical notes and colors: neither good nor bad, they simply are, and some we like better than others. I bet you never thought of emotions from such a neutral perspective. Of course, there are feelings you go out of your way to experience, such as satisfaction and joy, and others you might not be so crazy about, such as disappointment and fear. But because of how emotions make you feel, you've unconsciously made the erroneous decision to welcome only the ones that cause you to feel "good," and you cold-shoulder the ones that cause you to feel "bad." You've confused the function of feelings with their effect on you, but in truth they all have the same raison d'être: to give you information about how to negotiate this world in order to have the best possible life.

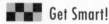 **Get Smart!**

How do you feel about experiencing intense emotions? What's your typical reaction to emotions that cause you to feel uncomfortable? How will you remind yourself to view them neutrally, exclusively as information transmitters?

What Can I Do with My Feelings?

This is a question I'm asked regularly, and it speaks to a uniquely Western notion that taking action is the best approach to whatever ails us, the operative word here being *do*. Fact is, sometimes there is something to do with a feeling, and sometimes there isn't. If your father died two weeks ago and you're feeling extremely sad and want to bawl like a baby, that's natural and normal and there is nothing to *do* except whatever comes up for you. If your father died twenty years ago, and the anniversary of his death still throws you into a downward spiral that sends you to bed for a week, it's time to make adjustments so you'll experience less pain and remain more functional. My point is that how frequent, intense, and lasting the feeling or residue of feeling (recalling emotions via memory) is dictates whether you need to do anything with it.

Humans are creatures of habit and, therefore, we tend to settle into one way of acting or reacting even when it doesn't work particularly well for us. That's unfortunate, because flexibility is absolutely key to effective emotional management. Too many folks, troubled and nontroubled eaters alike, shut off their feelings automatically. They hurt, then deny or act in ways to numb their feelings and move on. That's the way they learned to cope with intense affect when they were children and didn't know any better. Alternatively, perhaps they have an inkling that shutting down isn't really beneficial but are terrified of experiencing emotions and determined to keep their distance.

However, avoiding feelings is not a great idea, because feelings have a function. Consider someone who mistreats you repeatedly. In order to let them know that either they must change or you will need to cut them out of your life, you first must acknowledge that they have hurt you. Without the recognition of hurt, you'd be the equivalent of emotionally deaf or blind. Emotions act as guides, but they're only effective if you pay attention to them the way you pay attention to your senses. When you poke your tongue at a tooth that's throbbing, the purpose of that pain is to tell you something is wrong. Conversely, when you take a whiff of roses and are enveloped in a lovely, heady scent, you're using your senses to tell you that something is bringing you pleasure.

One of the reasons we don't care for intense emotion is that it can easily and excessively dysregulate us. It's difficult to be zapped by a strong feeling and not have it shake you up internally. We call this effect emotional dysregulation — it knocks us off course, throws us for a loop, pulls the rug out from under us. However, it's the way we feel about and react to dysregulation that makes or breaks us, emotionally speaking. Rather than accept that we're momentarily (okay, sometimes a lot longer than momentarily) off-kilter, and that this is natural and normal, we try to reregulate ourselves immediately. If we just give ourselves a little time, our bodies and minds often move toward reregulation on their own. Instead, though, we rush off for a snack so it can perform its magic act. A better approach is to remind ourselves that it's okay to not always feel perfectly centered or calm, and that we'll regain our equilibrium in good time with the right practices. You'll read more about dysregulation and reregulation in chapter 6.

▰▰ Get Smart!

How do you know when you're emotionally dysregulated? What specific feelings cause this to happen? What experiences cause these feelings? How does food reregulate you? What else, other than eating, helps reestablish a comfortable stasis?

Dr. Taylor maintains that we don't *have* to extend an emotional response beyond ninety seconds. What she's saying is that initial affective pain gets triggered automatically on a physical level owing to our nervous system. That's because the pain has a purpose, which I'll get to in a minute. The radical implication here is that experiencing pain beyond the initial stab of ouch is, in a sense, our choice. I say radical because, when we're in the throes of distress, few among us recognize that we are actually going out of our way to prolong our agony.

But heartache feels so real and so involuntary, you may insist — you wound me, I bleed. It does feel that way. However, once the initial zap has come and gone, we're responding not to authentic distress but to a *memory* of the distress we've just been experiencing! We're responding to a recollection of the pain we experienced a moment ago, not the actual wounding, which is already history (though very recent), come and gone, over and done with. Once the initial sting of hurt lets up, instead of distancing ourselves from emotional distress we may circle back around and poke at and prod it until it starts in again. We tell ourselves: "It's not fair that I didn't get invited to Susie's dinner party! I invited her to mine." "How could he embarrass me in front of the whole department just for being a few minutes late? Like he's always on time." "Mom/Dad/Sister/Brother can be so cruel. I'm so hurt by what she [or he] said. Forget about my going to visit on Sunday."

Let's use my client's mutinous office situation to further illustrate this point. As he sat in my office talking about that awful moment of sheer terror decades before, when he had feared being exposed and branded a whistle-blower in his company, it was another gorgeous day in Sarasota, and he was gazing out my office window at the tangle of overgrowth that lets loose in a subtropical climate after rainy season. He was calm and related the story with moderate emotion.

Although he said he could *recall* feeling as if his goose were about to be publicly cooked some thirty years earlier in that staff meeting, he certainly wasn't having the intense emotional response he'd had back then. That's because his memory had stored the data about that occurrence separately from the affect that it generated. Of course, maybe two days or two weeks after the interaction, he could still painfully recall being nearly found out, but even then he couldn't possibly feel the intense waves of affect he had experienced *at the time they occurred.*

Why? Because our automatic reactions have a very precise and singular reason for being. They grab our attention with a wallop of sensation to warn us of perceived immediate or imminent danger so that we can avoid, prevent, or minimize it. Now hear this: *The purpose of emotions — their sole raison d'être — is to steer us away from pain and keep us safe.* In evolutionary terms, that means they zap us to help us live — and breed — another day. Put another way, they generate pain to try to help us in the long run. Pain is acute to signal a warning to never forget a situation that has the potential to threaten our lives. The importance of grasping this concept cannot be overstated.

Like everything else in life, pain has a function — as does pleasure — and that function is first and foremost to preserve and propagate the species. On the pleasure front, for example, the neurotransmitter dopamine gets triggered in our brains when we eat high-fat, high-sugar foods, because many millennia ago they provided us with the greatest sustenance in the ancient, nutrient-scarce world in which we lived. We also experience a blast of dopamine during orgasm, a nifty incentive to keep on procreating. Our biochemistry developed over time — through evolution — the ability to fine-tune our reactions to pleasure and pain in order to keep us keeping on as a species.

Pain serves this purpose rather well. When something hurts, we tend to avoid doing whatever we think will cause more of it. We associate pain with perceived harm to self, and that's why we often have to talk ourselves into going to the dentist or the doctor, who might "hurt" us in the short run to heal us in the long run. When we experience pain, the primitive part of our brain registers the occurrence sharply and deeply so that we'll recall it automatically in case we find ourselves in a similar situation in the future.

Why Do I Sometimes Still Feel Bad Long after I've Been Emotionally Wounded?

You're not alone in that. We all have this tendency. The question can be answered by taking the idea of "emotional pain as an alarm signaling a perceived threat" one step further. Then you'll understand what I mean when I say that emotional pain *after an event* is not a response to reality but to recalling the occurrence that caused it. Let's backtrack a minute, to be sure you understand this important point. Remember that emotional pain — betrayal, rejection, fear, loneliness — and physical pain are intended as automatic warnings to *do* something to ward off danger and protect yourself. Remember as well that, once the threat has passed, this warning no longer has a function. It loses its purpose when the threat is over, much as a signalman on a train track has nothing more to do after the caboose has passed him by. No need to wave those flags to alert the engineer about a steep incline, because the danger — and the train — are long gone.

Here's another example. If a lion rushed at you, you'd feel fear instinctively and immediately, which would mobilize your internal resources, enabling you to do something to prevent a mauling — duck, fight, run, hide. Comedian Richard Pryor had this brilliant routine about being frightened that says it all: "Feet, don't fail me now!" Isn't that more or less what you'd think if a lion charged at you? However, if the lion heard a sudden noise, stopped dead in its tracks, then hightailed it in the opposite direction from where you were standing and disappeared into the woods, your psychic alarm still might be clanging as the cortisol rush to energize you subsides. The cortisol rush subsides because, no longer having a function, alarm chemicals slowly stop being produced in your brain and circulated in your body as soon as they have served their purpose and you're out of danger.

Pain is a way of etching risk and threat into our brains. Remember, our biology is geared to thwart repeat performances of anything that puts us at perceived emotional or physical harm. So, down the road, having been charged by a lion (and scared out of your wits), it's likely that if you're at the zoo and you stroll past a lion in its cage rushing over to say hello, your heart may begin to race and fear may course through your body. That's because the memory of a lion almost mauling you years before comes instantly to the fore before you can realize that you're quite safe because you're outside the cage, not inside it with Leo the lion. There's no longer a need for psychic pain — in this instance imprinted as fright — to warn you of harm, but it happens anyway because the amygdala, where intense affect is stored, cannot distinguish between the initial unsafe situation, which happened years ago, and the current, strikingly similar situation in which you aren't in danger.

Returning once again to my whistle-blower-in-the-office anecdote in which my client feared being outed: it made sense for him to be scared at the time, but not for him to reexperience intense fear as he sat in my cozy office looking out at palm trees, Spanish moss, and giant scheffleras. There was no need for strong emotion to warn him of danger, because he was in no danger in the present. The danger had passed. So, he could choose to recall the visual and tactile impressions of the memory of the staff meeting (who was there, where he was sitting, what the room looked like, the time of day) without strong affective impression.

Of course, there are times when you want to review a previously threatening situation to make better sense of it or assess what you could have done differently, times when you want to access didactic or factual memory. You may wish to understand why your spouse left you, why you were bullied in school, or why your mother let your father beat her up. However, you can access the details of these memories without re-experiencing the emotional pain attached to them, by reminding yourself that the pain no longer has purpose because the event is over. Think of it this way: if you are safe now and feel fear, that fear goes with the memory that caused it in the first place.

Because pain is a signal to do something to make yourself safe, it's overkill to have it clanging an alarm when you're no longer in harm's way. You can stop this unnecessary alarm by using your cognitive abilities, the higher-functioning part of your brain that can think logically, to remind yourself that you are no longer at risk and are quite safe. For sure, you want your automatic pain-response system to do its job when you're in actual emotional danger, but *only* when you are. If pain is coming from memory, not reality, that's a false alarm and your warning system needs a mental rewire.

▰▰ Get Smart!

Put into your own words the function of emotional pain (explaining will help you remember it). Can you think of an experience in which you were perfectly safe but continued to feel distressed by emotional pain that was socked away in your memory? Can you see how the later experience was only a false alarm? What can you now say to yourself when you have this kind of faux reaction?

The reason I'm harping on this pain model is because much of the emotional discomfort we feel in the present isn't about the here and now at all. Our discomfort is a reaction to a memory triggered by a situation similar to one in which we had previously been in danger. Unfortunately, our amygdala, where intense memories are stored, can't filter itself or tell the difference between past and present circumstances. That's not in its job description. Rather, it senses threat and immediately begins releasing chemicals to snag our attention and alert us that we may be in danger. Its motto may as well be: "Watch out. Here we go again." That's when we need our higher-order brain structures to tease out whether there truly is danger in the present. Most of the time when we're reacting strongly to fear or upset, it's out of recall, not reality.

Here are some examples to illustrate my point. The fact that your wife is ignoring you and hanging out with her friends at a party may unconsciously trigger the neglect you felt as a child when your mother would have her friends over to visit and leave you all alone and insist you not bother her. Your boss chewing you out in front of a client may trigger how ashamed you felt when your father would attend your soccer games and yell insults at you in front of the coach and other players. Your neighbor dropping over at all hours of the day or night without being invited may trigger your memory of Grandma walking into your room, without knocking, whenever she felt like it, your privacy be damned.

Get the picture? Much of the time when we're upset in the here and now it's due to intense upset from the there and then. If you are to become skilled in managing your emotions, you can't ignore this cause-and-effect reaction. Instead, every time you feel a strong emotion, you'll want to stop and consider if *what you're experiencing is in proportion to the emotional danger you perceive*. Sometimes it is and sometimes it isn't, and it's essential to discern the difference so that you'll know how to respond.

What Can I Do When I Feel All Discombobulated Inside?

The answer to this question has several parts. First, you want to acknowledge your discombobulation and *identify* what you're feeling. Don't lump all your emotions together under the umbrella of hurt or upset. That would be like telling a friend you had a phone call from "someone" about "something." Of course, your friend would ask, "Well, who called and what did he say?" Be specific: you're feeling anxious, betrayed, inadequate, frustrated, rejected, ashamed, lonely, guilty, disappointed, helpless, enraged, or confused. Get the gist of it? The more specific you are, the more information you'll extract from the emotion, because — make no mistake — information is precisely what you're after.

Here's another dose of wisdom from Dr. Taylor, who advises us to be open to feelings from the here and now whenever they come, at whatever intensity we experience them. If we short-circuit them, we won't receive the full benefit of the message they're delivering. On the other hand, if we continue to stoke their fires, we'll end up holding on to discomfort unnecessarily and ruin the quality of our lives.

Sometimes, a feeling blasts you when you least expect it, but you know just what it is. Maybe you catch the guy you thought was your boyfriend while he's smooching your best friend and feel a stab of betrayal. Perhaps you hear that your brother is being sent overseas with a combat unit next week, leaving no time to say good-bye, and you feel a surge of fear and sadness in your gut. Alternatively, at times you may sense a vague emotion erupting and want to work to identify it. For example, say your colleagues all ducked out for a drink at 4:20 and you're left to meet a 5 PM deadline alone. You know that what they did doesn't sit right with you, but you're not exactly sure what you're feeling, until suddenly a wave of abandonment washes over you. You feel like Little Miss Muffet stranded on her tuffet.

What about Feelings about My Feelings?

Clients often share with me how they feel about their painful feelings, which can be summed up as: not so good. I then ask them why they need to feel anything about their emotions. Why can't they simply experience a primary feeling, then not have it anymore, game over? Usually secondary emotions (feelings about feelings) are evaluative and judgmental about whether the initial, or primary, feeling is good or bad, tolerable or intolerable, acceptable or unacceptable. I'm not talking here about having two feelings at the same time — say, joy that your best friend got a new job and sadness that it's two states away from you. The secondary feelings that crop up are more than likely shame or guilt. You may feel shame that, for example, you're angry at a coworker who's gone out of his way to be nice to you but who recently ticked you off, or you may feel guilt for wanting to stay home when it's snowing outside and your kids want to go sledding.

Try your best to experience a feeling fully when it first comes around. Just showing up for it is all you have to do. Shoo away secondary feelings of guilt or shame and stick with the initial emotion until it subsides. Examples of primary emotions are as follows: shock at not getting a job for which you thought you were a shoo-in; sadness that your cat died; confusion over whether you should stay married after you find out your spouse has cheated on you; grief at being told you cannot bear children; loneliness after moving halfway around the world to where you don't know anyone; or guilt because, after having a fight with your neighbor, you came home and yelled at your children.

Stay with the feeling without trying to extend or curtail it, and by all means, ignore judgments about it. When the most intense part of the experience is over, congratulate yourself on a job well done, one that at times feels a bit like charging around on a bucking bronco. If you stayed in the saddle, give yourself a round of applause.

Get Smart!

Do you often have secondary feelings about your primary feelings? Which emotions tend to generate a judgment from you? Is that judgment necessary or simply habit? What can you say when you judge your feelings that will allow you to remain curious, open, and neutral about them?

What Skills Are Needed for Effective Emotional Management?

There are several ways to slice this pie. We could say that what's needed are two major emotional skill sets to keep yourself emotionally regulated: the ability to contain feelings *and* the ability to expand feelings as necessary. This involves trusting people enough to express and share emotional upset, take in honest feedback, and feel supported while also possessing various internal methods of responding to emotions when you're alone or it's not beneficial to express them. This is a tall order, to be sure, but doable. When handling emotions, many folks pick one approach only, and maybe you do, too. You may fear burdening others or not trust them sufficiently to be vulnerable in their presence, so you hold in emotions until you're ready to burst — or binge. Or perhaps you easily become overwhelmed with intense affect and call every friend in your iPhone desperately hoping that *someone* will say *something* to make you feel better.

Essentially, the goal is to comfortably ask for help and to also do all right without it. The ability to solicit and enjoy support comes from a mind-set in which you believe that many, most, or at least some people will understand what you're feeling and will empathize with you and validate what's going on within you. Being able to seek help also means you don't believe the ridiculous notion that you *should* be able to manage intense emotions on your own. Likewise, knowing you have substantial emotional competence makes you feel strong and capable on your own and leads you to solicit help only when it's necessary. No surprise, huh, that you're looking for a balance of resources, within and without?

Another way to view what Harvard author Daniel Goleman, PhD, calls "emotional intelligence" is to assess your skill at engaging and disengaging with emotion when necessary. If you're in the middle of a job interview and a disagreement you had with your daughter that morning pops into your head, you want to be able to shelve it for the moment, rather than spend time right then figuring out who was at fault. If you continue to ruminate days later about your quarrel after you and your daughter have made up, you want to be skilled at a technique called mindfulness in order to merely observe, rather than engage with this particular memory that will kick up a whole lot of affective dander that is best left to settle and dissipate.

At the opposite end of the spectrum, it's also vital that you fully engage with and experience emotions when they plop themselves on your doorstep. For example, say you've planned a night out with a friend, and he calls at the last minute to say he's too tired or busy, and this is something he's done umpteen times before. This is a perfect moment to connect with your emotions, which are likely to include feeling disappointed, neglected, hurt, and misused. What vital information you're getting about the quality of your relationship with this so-called friend! You want his thoughtlessness to register deeply so that you can avoid getting hurt in the future. Perhaps you'll want to talk with him about his unacceptable behavior or even end the friendship.

▉▉ Get Smart!

Do you commonly either contain your feelings or expand them? That is, do you feel you must handle them alone, or do you incline toward almost totally relying on others to help you reregulate yourself? Which skill would you like to improve, and how will you do this? Can you feel emotions deeply in the moment and absorb their wisdom? Do you fear and avoid your feelings? Do you dwell on and get lost in them beyond what's necessary in order to sort out and overcome distress?

Will I Ever Improve at Soothing Myself without Food?

It's true that emotional eaters generally turn to food when their feathers are ruffled, and they don't practice more effective ways to smooth them out. There are several reasons for this. Studies on temperament reveal that some people may actually be more emotionally sensitive than others, owing to genetic tendencies involving neurotransmitter imbalances, among other things. We all recognize that some folks are simply born sunnier and more upbeat than others. That's hard wiring. Moreover, how our childhood role models, primarily our caretakers, soothed themselves is a strong predictor of how we'll soothe ourselves. Our parents can't teach us what they didn't know how to do.

If Dad stormed off in a huff to his basement workshop and Mom made a beeline for the refrigerator every time they had a tiff, we see two approaches to handling emotions — neither of which shows great competence or effectiveness. I will say that, culturally, women seem to reach out and men seem to withdraw, and this is part of our evolutionary heritage. In the days of the cave dwellers, out on a hunt for food with the guys was not the time or place to be complaining about the kids misbehaving and driving you crazy. How much easier it was for women sitting around the fire tending to those very children to start gabbing about them. Sadly, since cave dweller times, the strong, silent male and the overly emotional female have remained cultural stereotypes, and we, as both children and adults, absorb their characteristics and frailties without realizing it.

Moreover, when you're upset, it's so easy these days to turn to food that people often don't even try to develop effective skills to cope with feelings and comfort themselves. To do so means unlearning "I-feel-therefore-I-eat" behaviors and acquiring skills that involve a good deal of practice. The truth is, although you might wish to have these self-calming skills, the issue is not about desire but about how hard you're willing to work to become proficient at them. They absolutely will not become part of your repertoire simply because you lay yourself down to sleep and pray for them. Rather they will become more integral to your coping strategies the more you put attention on and repeat them.

The problem with acquiring these skills instead of grabbing a sweet or other treat is that at first you may not find them particularly helpful. The frustration of learning new methods of self-care can generate hopelessness and helplessness. You might even believe that you'll never learn how to comfort yourself or relax without food even if you were to live three lifetimes. You may practice these skills a few times and give up, or you may use them at times and turn to food at other times, so that you're not making true progress. Remember, mastery comes from doing the new behavior more times than the old one — many, many more times, I might add. The truth is, if you do any behavior often enough, you will lay down new neural pathways in your brain and it will become habit.

Here are some basic ways to calm down and soothe yourself without food. This list is not meant to be exhaustive; there are scores of books (including my *Food and Feelings Workbook*) that can give you detailed advice on the subject. There's no shortage of helpful information out there to be gained through psychotherapy (individual or group), support groups, workshops, podcasts, message boards, and even apps such as my free Facebook app, APPetite.

That said, to unwind or comfort yourself you can learn and practice the following to replace unwanted eating:

- In the physical arena: To relax your body, drink a cup of tea; take a bath or shower; close your eyes and take a nap; do neck rolls; take a walk, swim, or ride a bike; get up and dance or do kickboxing; do catlike stretches; sit quietly and visualize a happy scene from your life; walk the dog or play with the cat; practice yoga; do a relaxation progression from toe to head; massage your temples, scalp, or any tense spots on your body; get regular massages; garden or do light chores; rock in a chair or a hammock; or (my favorite) do deep breathing.

- In the sensual arena: To awaken your senses other than taste, light a scented candle and inhale the aroma; go outside and smell flowers or freshly mowed grass; play music you love; rub cream all over your body; immerse yourself in a book of photography or watch a video of exotic places; look through magazines that bring you visual pleasure; stroke a bunch of various soft fabrics; or pet the dog or the cat.

- In the mental arena: To relax by enlivening your thoughts and rejuvenating your energy, browse through a joke book; check out humorous videos; watch a funny sitcom; engage in a hobby or passion; read a book that's a page-turner; surf the web; check your email; turn on the history, science, or nature channel; or teach yourself something new.

- In the emotional arena: For self-soothing, say compassionate, kind, caring things to yourself; reread a loving letter from someone; develop and repeat a mantra about your lovability; give yourself a hug; curl up in a fetal ball; cry; call someone who will help you feel better; tell yourself that your mood or the crisis will pass; if you made a mistake, remind yourself that you're allowed to make them; acknowledge that you're feeling bad, but remind yourself that this doesn't mean there's anything wrong with you; picture a strong, bright candle within you that burns with self-love; or write a love letter to yourself.

Want an instant fix for stress or distress? Don't reinforce what you're feeling. Instead, shift your self-talk to how you *wish* to feel, not whatever emotion you're experiencing. Some examples:

- If you're starting to feel overwhelmed, the last thing you want to say is, "Man, I am so overwhelmed. I feel awful. I can't stand this feeling." Instead, tell yourself, "I can handle this. It isn't so bad. I'm competent and will manage."

- If you're feeling frustrated, steer clear of messages like "This is too hard. I can't do it. I hate when I can't do things." Instead, say, "Oh, this isn't so bad. I'm getting the hang of it. Soon I'll succeed."

- If you're standing in front of the mirror hating your body, avoid insisting, "I look terrible. I'm so fat, I can't bear looking at myself." Instead, shift to: "My eyes are great, so blue and sparkly. I love that my body is getting healthier." (Then, step away from the mirror!)

- If you're falling into loneliness, mind that you don't make it worse by telling yourself, "I'll never have any friends. I'm just not good at relating to people. Who'd want to be my friend anyway, because I'm such a loser." Instead, show some self-compassion and offer yourself these kind words: "I have had friends, and I have some now. I can learn to feel more comfortable with people and have a circle of friends that feels just right to me."

- If your anxiety is skyrocketing, never, ever let these words pass your lips: "I'm feeling so panicky. I may be having a panic attack, and I don't know what I'll do. I can't bear feeling so anxious and out of control." Instead, soothe yourself by saying, "I'm fine and my anxiety is receding. I'm feeling calmer, cooler, and more collected." (For a really quick fix, do this while practicing deep breathing.)

You likely will have to try out many of these techniques to discover what works for you. Some options will bomb, and others will make you feel better only after you've practiced and are used to doing them. Find one or two strategies in each arena. Remind yourself that food is not the answer, and that you'd need to develop emotional management skills even if you didn't have an eating problem. Everyone needs them! Don't come down hard on yourself for not having these competencies. Merely remind yourself that all adults are learning life skills and that's how the game is played.

▰▰ Get Smart!

If you'd never heard of food, what would you do to soothe yourself or relax? Which of the alternatives to eating for de-stressing or comforting yourself that I've just described have you tried? If they didn't work, why not? What will you do to develop effective emotional management strategies? What stands in your way? What will help you succeed?

Skill Boosters

1. Notice whether an upset is mild, moderate, or intense. Rather than judge it, be curious about it and acknowledge, identify, and experience it with calmness and the certainty that it will

yield important information about your life. Consider it a text message from you to you.

2. If you're afraid of experiencing emotions intensely, sink more deeply into them by assigning a number to an emotion you're feeling, to identify how deeply you're feeling it. Use a scale of 1 to 5, with 1 representing superficial engagement, 3 representing substantial engagement, and 5 indicating complete engagement. If you're at 1, move yourself to 2, then 3. If you're at 3, move yourself to 4, then 5.

3. Practice being curious about and compassionate with your emotions. If you slip into judgment, use mindfulness to notice this has happened and return to curiosity and compassion.

4. If you tend to always run to others for comfort when you're in emotional distress, rather than building effective coping resources within, see how far you can get while comforting yourself on your own.

5. If you tend to clam up, stay private, or lick your wounds alone when you're in emotional turmoil, reach out to a trusted someone. It doesn't matter if you're uncomfortable. That only means you're doing something unfamiliar.

6. Recognize feelings associated with stress — frustration, inadequacy, a sense of being overwhelmed — and talk yourself down from them. Practice extreme relaxation.

7. If you tend to ruminate and go over the same miseries again and again, remind yourself that your strong reaction is not from the present, that you're caught in a memory, and that replaying it will change nothing. Ground yourself in the present by reconnecting to your body in the current time and place and breathing deeply.

8. Every day, practice effective life skills from the arenas listed earlier. Don't wait until you're in a crisis. You must do these new activities *every single day* for new neural pathways to form. In fact, building a preventive routine is your best bet for keeping yourself emotionally regulated.

9. Stop during the day to notice whether you're emotionally

regulated or dysregulated, and be aware of which people, interactions, and events generate each state. Before engaging in an activity that would typically dysregulate you, or before being around a person who may do so, prepare yourself by relaxing and recognizing your concern. Work on reregulating yourself as soon as you've finished the activity or are away from dysregulating people.

10. If you have the urge to eat when you're not hungry, know that your desire is not for food. Ask yourself what you're feeling, and stay with it until you find the right approach to address whatever you're feeling (for example, sit with it, notice but don't engage with the feeling, de-stress, and so on).

In chapter 4, you'll learn how to avoid living in the past or future and stay anchored to the present.

CHAPTER 4

Living Consciously

I'm Conscious Only of Wanting to Go Unconscious!

Humans have a funny orientation toward life. Although their heads remain securely attached to their bodies, their minds often drift off into the past or leap ahead into the future. You know what I mean. You're at your son's birthday party serving cake to all the four-year-olds, and instead of enjoying the moment, you're wondering what their parents will say about your party after they've gone. Will they think the games were fun and that your home was attractive, or will they be appalled that the cake was store bought and not homemade, and wonder why you couldn't have been more creative with the decorations?

Or, in an equally possible scenario, you might be doling out cake slices to those four-year-olds while agonizing about the fight you had on the phone that morning with your mother, who wanted to come to the party but didn't want to drive in the rain. She was angry that you wouldn't pick her up and take her home, and you're feeling guilty for saying no because you had so much to do. Although you're trying to have a good time on your son's behalf, you're so lost in your own thoughts of past and future that you can barely figure out who has cake and who doesn't.

This is not what we call living consciously — that is, with intent and awareness and a focus on the here and now. That only happens when all your energy — mental and physical — is directed toward the present moment. Of course, no one does this conscious-living thing perfectly, so the idea isn't to always be grounded in the present, but to be there as often as possible, certainly more often than not; know when you're slipping out of it; and be able to bring yourself back as quickly as possible.

The goal is to stay intentionally conscious except when you purposely want to shut off your mind and attention and give yourself a large or small mental vacation. Dysregulated eaters are often confused about when to intentionally focus on the reality at hand and when to zone out — what Geneen Roth, an eating-disorders author and educator, calls "going unconscious." Because focusing on and tuning out the present are mutually exclusive mental states, we can't do both at once. Consequently, not being clear on which choice to make can lead to a paradoxical state of becoming hyperconscious of food and craving it in order to surrender consciousness through eating. This contradiction is complicated, and I'll talk more about it in a moment. For now, suffice it to say that dysregulated eaters need to learn the skill of staying mentally in the present both with food and in other areas of life unless they have a valid purpose for intentionally thinking about the past or future.

◼◼◼ Get Smart!

Do you live consciously in the here and now, or are you on autopilot most of the time? Have you tried to live more consciously? What more could you do to make this happen? What's the difference in your eating habits when you're aware or unaware? What's the difference in your life when you are mindful or functioning on automatic?

Is It a Weird Kind of Magic Trick That We're Physically in the Present, Yet Manage to Mentally Disappear?

Yes, there is a kind of magic to thinking you're in the present while not being there mentally, or operating so automatically that you're unaware of being wherever you are. There are two ways we miss out on the here and now. Both are perfectly natural, human tendencies and cannot be entirely driven out of us like evil spirits. But with skill and practice, they can be limited in order to enhance our eating and our lives.

Living on Autopilot

When we live on autopilot, we're not necessarily dwelling on the past or catapulting our thoughts into the future. In fact, our minds are in a kind of netherworld, as if our brains have shifted, unbeknownst to us, into pause mode. We're not consciously thinking about other things, nor are we concentrating on what we're doing. If someone asks what we're thinking about, we might give her a startled look and laugh sheepishly. "I'm not sure," "Nothing really," or "I have no idea," we might say. Although we've disconnected our thinking from the present, we haven't really connected it to anything else either.

This experience often happens when you're doing routine tasks like mowing the lawn, ironing, or chopping vegetables. You're not cogitating on something else; in fact, you're not cogitating at all. Your body is definitely engaged in activity, but your mind isn't. This is not necessarily a negative occurrence. There's a distinct pleasure in doing repetitive tasks that demand little attention. They give your busy, weary mind a nice little break, perhaps the equivalent of taking an intentional catnap when you're tired in the middle of a hectic afternoon. When you purposely choose to shut off your mind and let your body do its thing, you may benefit greatly from the experience.

However, when you live on autopilot, whether you've intentionally chosen to or not, that's quite another thing. And this is often what dysregulated eaters do. They feel such pressure to get so many things done so perfectly that they whiz through the day without putting attention on any of them. If they're not zipping the kids to school, they're rushing off to work and racing through the day to get back to pick up the kids and throw together dinner. They do what they think they ought to do and miss out mentally on the actual experience of doing it. That's why at the dinner table when you ask your son how his day went, he says, "Mo-om, I told you all about it in the car on the way home. Weren't you listening?" Well, no, Mom, actually you weren't. In fact, you have no idea what was in your mind, except you seemed to have paid enough attention to driving to have ferried the kids home safely.

In *Care of the Soul: A Guide for Cultivating Depth and Sacredness in Everyday Life*, a book that sounds religious but is quite secular, author Thomas Moore shines a light on how little attention we pay to everyday life and how greatly we suffer for it. He teaches us to see each moment as sacred, as precious, as a building block of life. As Moore sees it, we want to be as fully engaged in washing dishes as in life's grander moments, as present to suffering as to joy, as eager to partake in the mundane, routine aspects of life as we are to experience the extraordinary, unique, mind-blowing ones.

This makes sense, since there are many more humdrum moments than astounding or exceptional ones. If we pay attention only to the "big events," then we miss most of what happens to us. However, if we treat every moment as worthwhile, with full engagement, we live more richly and fully. Dysregulated eaters often are bored with their lives and are constantly seeking stimulation because they're cut off from the now. Moore says that stimulation is right there in front of your face, in everything you do — brushing your teeth, paying bills, changing a lightbulb, getting your hair cut, mowing the lawn, lifting weights, or filling your car with gas — and I heartily agree with him.

By fading in and out of life, you miss so much and often feel unfulfilled, not because your life isn't interesting or full, but because you exhibit very little interest in or connection to it. And this lack of attentiveness to each and every aspect of life leaves you feeling empty and apathetic, creating a kind of ennui that too often makes you look to food for engagement and excitement. When you remain emotionally connected to everything you do, you continuously fill up in small ways, and you avoid the emptiness that might drive you to mindless eating.

Living in the Past or the Future

Obviously, you recognize that I'm not referring to time travel — which, as far as I know, is not possible. When I talk about living in the past or future, I expect you understand that I mean shifting mental awareness away from the present and recalling what's come before or anticipating what lies ahead. This is a mental process, not a physical act, and there's nothing wrong with thinking about the past or the future if we do it intentionally and purposefully.

There are lots of excellent reasons to deliberately call up memories. We enjoy reminiscing about earlier times because it brings us pleasure and is often a bonding experience if we do it with others we knew way back when. Even on a practical level, thinking about the past is important for, say, recalling how we did something at work that turned out well, so that we can repeat our success. Moreover, as the adage says, how can we know where we're going if we don't know where we've been?

What I'm talking about here is the act of purposely moving your attention from the present to what came before. On a biological level, that means using the parts of our brains that store both the data and the affect from our history, what we call memory. For instance, while one part of your brain has stored a great recipe for the rice pudding you used to make as a teenager for Thanksgiving, another has stowed away the loving feelings you had toward your now deceased brother, who used to love making rice pudding with you. When we intentionally seek out memories, we generally recognize why we're doing so. You want to pull up that rice pudding recipe because you're having the family over for Thanksgiving and everyone loves it. You want to linger over memories of your brother because that makes you feel closer to him and miss him less.

But what about those times you suddenly experience a memory, and it snatches you up and plunks you on its merry-go-round and won't let you off? Like the time you totally forgot what you were talking about while you were chairing a business meeting, and you couldn't seem to find the point you wanted to make anywhere in your notes. How embarrassing was that! It's awful to remember your shame, yet somehow you can't stop recycling the memory. Or perhaps you keep going over the decision you made to give notice at your job at the end of the month — you find yourself hurtling back and forth between being sure you are doing the right thing in leaving work you hate and being terrified that you'll never find another job and will be living on the streets after you get evicted from your apartment.

Being hijacked by memory is an unpleasant experience. There's a sense of helplessness, panic, and frustration, which feels a great deal like being trapped in a compulsion. This discomfort is often caused by the overwhelming drive to travel back in time and undo what you did. To use the example of your mind going blank while you're chairing a meeting, all you want to do is return to standing in front of your subordinates and colleagues and make every point in your notes clearly and fluidly, so that everyone at the table is roused to applause, so impressed are they with your knowledge and leadership skills. It's as if your memory isn't playing fair with you, leading you on by bringing up the experience as if it's actually happening, but not letting you intervene to make the story come out with a happier ending.

Regularly engaging in this kind of mental-do-over mind game can consume so much energy that you have little left over for the present. Moreover, every time we get seduced into believing that we can change what came before by ruminating on it, we are disappointed. What an awful way to live! More than likely, these frustrating feelings will keep your mood spiraling further and further down until you're so miserable that you don't care if food isn't a great choice. It feels better than being trapped in what seems like all the wrongness of your life.

Notice how different ruminating about your business situation is from intentionally trying to recall a piece of information or a pleasurable memory. In the former case, you feel powerless to make your life better, and in the latter you use your power to actually make it better. What is the singular difference between these forays into memory? In one, you're inadvertently slipping into a memory fragment with the unrecognized desire to engage in an impossible task: altering the past. In the other, you're expressly replaying a memory that's perfectly acceptable as is.

As unpleasant as it is to be trapped in the time warp of memory, it's equally agonizing to try to catapult yourself into the future, another mission impossible. You not only can't rewind and relive your life, but you can't fast-forward it either. Our efforts to do this spring from wanting to make sure life will be okay (actually, that we will be okay) when we get to wherever we think we're going. Here are some examples. You obsess about being a specific weight or clothes size three months from the present, the date of the cruise you've booked with your high school friends.

Or maybe you start planning out every minute of the visit your parents are making to your new house next weekend, so you can be sure they'll have a pleasant time. Or perhaps you can't stop thinking about your upcoming gastric bypass surgery.

Do you know what all these situations have in common? In each of them, you want to rush into the future and fix it, so that when you get there you'll be fine. Think about my explanation for a minute and see if it makes sense. Isn't that exactly what you do when you worry about the future? Your motivation is to think about it a lot *now* so it will be fine *when it happens*. It's as if your thoughts could somehow travel through space to a time that has yet to happen, solely to ensure that things will go swimmingly when you get there.

Please don't feel bad if you engage in this kind of mental gymnastics on a regular basis. It's another one of those quirks of being human. But it doesn't make your life work better, does it? And for sure, putting pressure on yourself to make life come out right doesn't help you eat "normally." Immersing yourself in expending that kind of mental energy fruitlessly on a regular basis depletes you and is a recipe for abusing food.

▰▰ Get Smart!

Do you ruminate about the past or worry incessantly about the future? Do you understand why you engage in these behaviors? How do they affect your eating?

Am I Doomed to Wander through Time Forever, or Can I Learn to Stay Put in the Here and Now?

Of course you can learn the skill of living consciously, as long as you're willing to make some alterations in your life and not expect to be perfectly present all the time. One of the best books on the subject of staying conscious is *The Power of Now: A Guide to Spiritual Enlightenment* by Eckhart Tolle. When I first heard of his book, it was already a huge bestseller, but I couldn't imagine reading an entire book whose premise was the need to pay attention to the present. The whole subject seemed so simplistic, and

I was sure I'd be bored silly reading the book. But one day I found it at a yard sale and said what the heck.

How wrong I was! It still seems almost impossible to believe that Tolle could say something interesting and enlightening on the subject of the power of now for nearly two hundred pages — and he's written a best-selling sequel! What he does is shift the way we think about the world, our place in it, our abilities, and how we want to live. So the question is: do you wish to live consciously? If so, then it is certainly within your grasp. If you don't, well, then, that's okay too; but by giving up this quest, you may not be able to shed your eating problems.

Assuming you do yearn for a more conscious existence, please recognize that the now is always waiting for you. You don't have to search for it. And when you're in it, you know it. We've all experienced that "awesome" sensation of being fully engaged. I felt it, powerfully, twice last night — while mesmerized by a gorgeous Florida sunset and then while sitting and watching TV and petting my cat. I was totally awestruck and wanted those moments to last forever.

These moments can happen to you anytime — while you're tinkering with the car, feeding your goldfish, getting ready for a tennis serve, cooking dinner, or cooing at your infant son. Whenever you lose track of time because you're absorbed in an activity or creative process, you're in the now. In these moments, something happens in our brains that brings us to attention and floods us with enormous pleasure. People have many names for this experience, and the ones I use are *peace* and *awe*. If you enjoy these feelings, you will certainly feel them more often when you spend more time in the here and now. No, not every moment will be filled with splendor and contentment, but you'll learn when you've left reality and how to get back there as you deepen your connection to life and to yourself.

▰▰ Get Smart!

Describe what it feels like to be wholly conscious. Name three reasons you would like to live more consciously.

How Do I Stay Conscious When I'm Pulled in So Many Directions and Don't Even Know When I Exit Reality?

One easy way to know that you've spaced out from reality is when you find yourself ruminating about the past or worrying about the future. Remember, you can't be in two places at once! To stay put, get in the habit of asking yourself routinely during the day: *Where am I?* Asking this question breaks the spell cast over you by wherever you've been hanging out. If you've been caught up in some memory fruitlessly trying to plot a better ending for it, you'll be automatically bounced back to the present by simply noticing where you are. If you've been attempting to stealthily creep up on the future to make it turn out all right, asking yourself where you are will yank you back to where you belong.

Here's an example. As I've been writing, I've been pulled back into the memory of a bit of tension in a group I belong to. A member took one of my comments personally and blamed me for hurting her feelings. Although I recognized that she was only trying to make herself feel better, her snarky comment kept snagging my attention away from writing this book. I'd get a few sentences down, then find myself lost in thought about how this interaction might affect the group as a whole, or how I'll handle the situation if she continues blaming me for her insecurities. This jumping back and forth from past to present to future has not been helping me get this chapter written and, moreover, has all but ruined the deep pleasure I find in writing, which usually completely captures my attention and energy. That's because writing is a very now experience!

So, every time I found myself drifting backward or propelling myself forward, I noticed the fact and returned myself to the written word. The more I did this, the less often I mentally wandered, until I stopped it completely when I was halfway through this chapter. Of course, I could have stepped away from my computer and taken a break while I considered what happened in the group and how I might respond were it to happen again, but that would have given too much power to the situation. There are times, though, that this would be the appropriate choice when something is bothering me.

The point is to break your unconscious connection to any point in time except the current moment. Consciousness awakens when you cut the cord to anywhere but now, and you cut the cord by seeking consciousness. After practicing this process until it feels natural, your mind will respond by not drifting off so often; and even if it does drift, you're far more likely to notice that you've shifted your attention and you'll readjust your mental sights more quickly.

Another way to stay with or return to the present is to use your body and your senses. Try stamping your feet or singing a song when you're in the middle of dredging up some awful memory you're trying to refashion or you're scouting the future for some disaster you're struggling to avert. What happens? Physical activity brings you right back to the present. This is why meditation is so powerful in the way it uses the breath. Paradoxically, breathing is a process that we are usually not conscious of — and that's all well and good. However, attending to the breath works wonders for bringing ourselves back whenever our minds have busted open the barn door and galloped off.

One of the best ways to stay out of memory, except when you have a reason to go there, is to understand the attraction it has for you. This process reminds me of how overeaters, when bored, will troll their refrigerators and kitchen cabinets for food. You know what I mean: how you suddenly stop what you're doing, fling open the refrigerator door, and poke around for something to eat, until you finally realize there's nothing you really want and return to whatever you were doing. That's what happens with memory. Sometimes we simply find ourselves there for no good reason. One minute we're in reality and the next, poof, we're being left at the altar, asked to resign from our job, standing at the crematorium during Mom's funeral, or lying in that lumpy hospital bed with both our legs in casts.

Why, we need to ask ourselves, are we missing out on the precious present and creating misery for ourselves? Of course, there is no logical answer to this question. We don't do it for any beneficial reason, but we might do it because we think we ought to. Maybe we're still processing the shame of being left at the altar, the panic at losing our job, the guilt of not being around when Mom died, or the helplessness of being stuck in bed unable to walk. In that case, we may think that returning to the memory will help us work through what happened. It might, but only if we are consciously choosing to think about the past in order to learn from it. It won't help a whit if we've slipped into a memory trance and have no idea why we're wandering around in a self-imposed nightmare.

Think about learning how to swim. There's a huge difference between falling or being pushed into a lake and intentionally jumping in because you want to take the plunge. The first situation leaves you feeling frightened and helpless, while the second might well lead to pleasure. If you think of memory in this light, you'll want to spend time in it only if it has important or relevant information to cough up.

The antidote to straying from consciousness into thoughts of the future is to understand what you're seeking in this process. As I've said, when you worry, you go over dozens of scenarios in your mind to try to nail down every detail, to put everything in order to ensure that when you arrive at some not-now time, all will be well. The important question is why you have this desperate drive. The answer is that you believe you'll be fine only if all is well, and that you won't be fine if it isn't.

Let this concept sink in for a minute. Isn't it true you fear that if all is not well in the future, then the applecart that will be upset will have your name on it? What are you really afraid will happen if you don't get into the college of your choice, find the right job or the right partner (or any partner at all!), finish all your errands, clean your house, have a child that turns out the way you want, make your flight, lose a certain amount of weight, spend more time with your kids, or live out all your dreams?

You're worried that you'll feel distress and unhappiness. Put another way, you're worried that you won't feel fine. So, let's follow this line of thinking. You're in the present and are expending an inordinate amount of time and energy making sure that you'll be fine at some distant date. Does that not seem a bit pointless? Does that not seem nigh impossible? How can we ever ensure, no matter how much we agonize and overplan, that life will be as we wish it to be? We might be able to if we were the only ones living on the planet, but maybe not even then. After all, there are always Mother Nature and Father Time with which to contend.

Please understand that doing something now can never, ever ensure that we'll be fine in the future. That is an impossibility, so you might as well cross that wish off your list. Am I saying that this means we can never be okay with what happens? That's a horrid thought and definitely not the point I'm trying to make.

There is a way to be fine in the future, and it's grounded in living consciously today. The only way we can guarantee we'll be fine in the future is to make sure we're fine today and every day thereafter. Try this on for size: If you're embedded only in the present and do your utmost to make yourself feel fine every moment of every day, you can't help but be fine in the future, which is the now that hasn't happened yet. After all, why wouldn't you do your best to be fine all the time? It's far more pleasant than not feeling fine, isn't it? I mean, if you had a choice to make yourself feel fine or not fine, which would you pick? You'd pick *fine*, of course.

And that, dear reader, is my point — you know you'll be fine in the future because your way of living is to always consciously work on feeling fine in the present. Feeling fine doesn't just happen — although some people are born with a tendency to be more upbeat, optimistic, and resilient than others, and still other folks have had awful things happen to them that make feeling fine more difficult. We make ourselves feel fine no matter what happens because, well, why wouldn't we do that?

As it happens, the way to be fine now and forever is to be conscious of how you feel in the moment. Consciousness of the present not only anchors you to it but also keeps you from a futile endeavor: worrying about the future. Some helpful advice: Make conscious decisions in the now that enable you to prepare for the future as much as anyone can prepare, and know that you can always choose to make yourself feel okay.

When I explain this process to clients or students in workshops, at this point I get a most useful question: Okay, so how *do* I make myself feel fine? If you were thinking this question, slap a gold star on your forehead, because it means you understand that you can make choices when you're conscious. For exactly how to make yourself feel better when things don't work out, when you're disappointed or hurt, I refer you to chapter 3, on emotions.

Just remember that the way to take care of your emotions is to remain conscious — that is, to be present to reality, moment by moment. In fact, in the present is the only place you can tend to your emotions. You can't change the ones that you've already felt, nor can you alter the ones you have yet to feel, no matter how much you brace yourself for them. All you can do with emotions is work with whatever you feel at the moment.

Here's an effective way to stay conscious through mindfulness. Think of thoughts as trains, and think of your mind as a train station. If you never travel by train, recall a time when you took trains or buses regularly. Did you have a certain train that took you to work or back home? When other trains stopped at the station, did you get on or let them pass? Of course, you simply watched them go by and waited for the train that would take you to your destination.

Imagine thoughts as being like that. Why engage with a thought that isn't going to take you where you want to go? If it's taking you back to some misery in your life — a failed exam, a stupid comment that hurt someone's feelings, a time you gravely disappointed yourself or others — let it go by. If it's headed for some anxiety-provoking place in your future — knee surgery, a family visit that's bound to be tense, a long overdue appointment with your doctor, or a meeting with your child's principal — let it go by, too. Hop only onto trains that are going where you want to go, to sunny, delightful places where you really want to spend emotional time!

▰▰ Get Smart!

What are the signs that you've left the present and are ruminating about the past? What are the signs that you've left the present and are worrying about the future? What is your specific plan for staying conscious? How will you feel fine?

If I'm Always Paying Attention in and to the Moment, When Do I Give My Brain Time Off for Good Behavior?

An excellent question. The way you give your brain a rest is to make a conscious choice to take time out. You decide that you've been paying a great deal of attention to minding the kids, taking care of your sick mother, tending to your overworked partner, or busting your butt at your job, and you give yourself explicit permission to chill out. You don't aim to do everything perfectly, expect to be all things to all people, push yourself beyond what's healthy, or tune out your feelings of stress or exhaustion. You observe that you're starting to feel tired and cranky and would benefit from a break.

Living consciously doesn't mean never relaxing or letting loose. Au contraire! It's the precise path to making the right choice at the right time. In my experience, dysregulated eaters do the opposite. They tend to go overboard and never, or rarely, give themselves permission to wind down, and therefore they seek the release they yearn for in mindless eating. Some of them sleepwalk through the rest of their lives as well, while others are so hypervigilant that they can't ever let loose.

When you live consciously, you choose pleasures and pastimes that are beneficial for you mentally and physically. You don't just fall into doing things because someone else is doing them, or because you've always done them. That would be the antithesis of living consciously. Rather, you notice the activities that put your brain on pause in a healthy way. What you're looking for — and there will be more about this subject in chapter 9 — are ways to zone out that leave you proud of yourself, not ashamed. You could come home from work and get drunk every night, which would definitely numb your brain, but you wouldn't feel too swell physically or mentally once the booze wore off. Food or drugs would have a similar outcome.

The truth is that dysregulated eaters don't practice turning off their brains in healthy ways. In my experience, many of them have neurotransmitter imbalances that make it difficult for them to easily chill out or perk up. The chemicals that normally have these effects aren't working very well for them, so they grab whatever seems to work, which is often food — and when I say *food*, I mean carbohydrates, because carbohydrates have inhibitory, anxiolytic, or excitatory, dopamine-generating properties. Unfortunately, people with biochemical imbalances must work extra hard to find healthy activities to change their moods.

Another way of talking about living consciously is to say we live mindfully. I find it sadly ironic that in order to be more mind*ful* of food, dysregulated eaters often need to become more mind*less* in other areas of life. Sometimes they're so vigilant about doing things right (or, worse, perfectly) everywhere else that the only time they feel they can let loose is while eating. So many dysregulated eaters keep themselves on a tight leash, never getting a chance to let it all hang out. By a *tight leash*, I don't mean they consciously make well-informed choices for themselves at every moment. I'm talking about worrying so much about others' approval, and about doing things just so, that anything that doesn't contribute to those outcomes falls by the wayside.

Living consciously means trying to be present to every minute, and not being obsessively attached to future outcomes — to success or to avoiding someone else's displeasure down the line. It means not ruining your current enjoyment by feeling guilt, shame, or remorse. These emotions are the antithesis of enjoying the here and now. Be most connected to what's at your feet, not to what's down the road those feet are traveling on. Of course, you always want to keep in mind where you're heading, and there's nothing wrong with planning for the future. But you don't want to keep your eyes glued to it so that you miss the reality at hand.

Dysregulated eaters use food in a paradoxical way in terms of consciousness. On the one hand, they can be more or less oblivious (depending on the person, circumstance, and level of awareness) to what they're eating. I recall that, at times, in my world-class binge-eating days, I ate boxes and bags of foods I barely tasted. Yet at other times, I prolonged and savored every excessive mouthful as if it were the last bite of food I'd ever take. Although much nonhunger eating is totally mindless, some of it throws dysregulated eaters into a general hyperawareness of food — that is, their desire for it is intense, which drives thoughts of anything else out of their minds, while the actual eating experience is an unconscious or only vaguely conscious one. It's as if, when they finally arrive at the actual eating experience, their brains can finally shut off — which is what they wanted to do in the first place. My take: it's often the idea of food that dysregulated eaters yearn for, not the food itself.

▚ Get Smart!

What do you do consciously to turn off your mind? Are these behaviors effective and healthy? Is it difficult to give yourself permission to let go and tune out? What emotions get in the way? Make a list of healthy ways to "go unconscious" that don't involve eating or thinking about food or weight.

In sum, in order to gain skills to live consciously, you have to know when you slip out of being conscious and how to reground yourself in the present. It's also helpful to know why you're tempted to not meet the moment as is. Maybe it's unpleasant to think about being single, and you'd rather daydream endlessly about the coworker you have a crush on, who's shown no discernible romantic interest in you. Maybe you, as a parent, spend so much time doubting the decisions you've made about your children that you have no energy left to enjoy your kids in the present. Finally, perhaps you're so hell-bent on making the future right that you forget to experience the now.

By slowing down and focusing all your senses on the present moment, you can live more consciously. At any time of the day, ask yourself what you see, hear, smell, and feel through touch. When you find yourself racing through the day, intentionally slow down or stop for a moment and ask, What's the rush? Rather than transitioning from one task directly to another, pause between tasks and take a few delicious deep breaths. Ah, there, now you're living consciously.

Skill Boosters

1. When you awaken, take three long, deep breaths and set your intention to live consciously all day.

2. Before you go to sleep, assess how you did in your effort to stay conscious that day. Be curious, not judgmental. Note when you were thrilled to notice you were conscious and engaged in the moment, and when you observed yourself slipping into memory or galloping off into the future.

3. Make a list of your major worries and prioritize them. Does worrying improve life? If you gave up worrying, what would happen for better or for worse? Write down three ways to be less anxious.

4. Identify memories you return to repeatedly as if you could have a do-over, and make a point of avoiding them by using the train metaphor. Remember, board only the trains that will take you to a destination you want.

5. Note when you're most conscious during the day — morning, afternoon, or evening — and in what circumstances. What enhances or hinders consciousness?

6. Take a mindfulness-meditation class.

7. Identify and practice one to three activities that keep you conscious and in the moment, and engage in them as often as you can. (Scientific studies tell us that being in nature is an especially soothing and centering experience.)

8. The next time you have an urge to eat when you're not hungry, observe your desire to be mindless, and find something to do to fill that need. Or, if you're bingeing, pull yourself out of unconsciousness and focus your full attention on what you're doing, without judging it. Tell yourself, "I love you."

9. Read books on mindful eating, and put signs up around your dining area to remind yourself to stay conscious of food — "How hungry am I? Am I enjoying my food? Slow down and chew! Am I still hungry, or am I done?" Ask intimates to gently point out when you are not living consciously. Keep a journal of conscious living.

10. Use a timer, and see if you can stay conscious and alert while thinking of nothing, without your mind drifting to other thoughts. Practice increasing the amount of time you can do this.

11. Learn and practice ways to self-soothe and use positive self-talk, so that you're always moving toward feeling fine.

In chapter 5, you'll learn how to enjoy interdependent and intimate relationships.

CHAPTER 5

Building and Maintaining Relationships

I Already Have a Great Relationship... with My Refrigerator!

Undoubtedly, at one time or another, you have thought of food as your best friend. It's there for the taking — or it's not more than a brief walk or car ride away — in all its glory, just waiting for you to pick it up for a hot date. Unlike certain people, food gives its all to you, and you perceive it as devoting itself completely to making you feel better. It has no needs of its own and offers no rebuffs or judgments. It lets you use it for pretty much whatever you please, and it never complains.

But if food were a true friend, you wouldn't be reading this book. I don't know where the idea of "food as friend" began, but it really is silly, when you think of what the term *friend* means. Friends have our back, protect us from self-delusion, offer their wisdom, and want the best for us. Food may be a comfort, but it's never a friend.

Yet it's understandable that we may be drawn to it when true friends or intimates are not readily available — or when we lack a nurturing self to take care of us. Problems arise when you come to believe that food is better than people at helping you cope with life, you dream and fantasize about eating rather than enjoy real relationships, and you give up being with people in order to be with food. Sadly, you probably have had the experience of hanging out with friends or family, or even a date, and not having a bad time, when seemingly out of the blue, food cravings erupt even though you're not hungry. Maybe last night's leftovers are in the

85

fridge, calling out to you, or maybe you have a vision of swinging by a fast-food joint and grabbing some takeout. Suddenly, the people around you seem to fall out of focus, and every fiber of your being is screaming to get *out of where you are* and to cozy up to a sweet or other treat. That's how it goes when cravings overpower our food-warped minds.

Even the idea of having a *relationship* with food is pretty bizarre, because we usually save the term for interactions in which there's an exchange, a give-and-take. Truth is, you're hardly having a "relationship" with food. You're using it (ineffectively, I might add) to meet your needs. If you want to become skilled at building and maintaining relationships, you'll need to give up the idea that you have one with things like Pop-Tarts, Doritos, and pizza. Remember, Ben, Jerry, and Mrs. Fields are someone's friends, but not yours. People who are skilled at enjoying relationships might enjoy Ben and Jerry or Mrs. Fields, but they don't mistake them for their best buds.

▪▪▪ Get Smart!

Do you think of food as a friend? List the ways in which it isn't a friend to you.

Genuine relationships give you so much more than food can or ever will. When you turn to food, you're seeking comfort, validation, quality companionship, empathy, understanding, fun, laughs, stimulation, excitement, and nurturance; you want to feel loved and valued. But while you may not have received these things from many folks in your life, this doesn't mean that you, as a human renting space on the planet, don't need and deserve them — or that you can't get them from people. With practice, you will.

What If I'm Not Great at Building and Maintaining Relationships, but I'm Super at Using Food to Make Myself Feel Better?

Learning a skill begins by admitting you know very little about a subject. So, you're in the right place, at the starting line. And you'll progress from here. Let's first figure out why you haven't been terrific at developing or holding on to relationships. After all, there must be a reason. The following questions will help.

1. What were your relationships with your parents like?
2. If you had siblings, what kind of relationships did you have with them?
3. How did your parents relate to each other?
4. How did family members relate to each other?
5. Did you feel loved and lovable as a child, that your boundaries were honored, and that you were respected, precious, and special?
6. Were your parents skilled at forming relationships outside the family? Did they have close, loving friendships and good relationships with their families?
7. While growing up, did you have solid friendships with classmates, kids in your neighborhood, teammates, or cousins?
8. Did you grow up in a stable community, or did you move from one place to another so that you had to make — and leave — friends over and over, and it was difficult to maintain ongoing relationships?
9. Were you shy or self-conscious around, or afraid of, other people, or were you bullied or teased a great deal as a child or adolescent?
10. Were you prevented or discouraged by your parents from making close friendships outside the home?

I hope these questions get you thinking about what modeling and instruction you received while growing up, which we might as well call Relationships 101. If you have trouble with closeness, you probably had a number of things going on in childhood. The first is that you may have had poor role models — parents with weak interpersonal skills who therefore couldn't teach you what you needed to know. If they didn't take much interest in you, or took too much interest and didn't give you sufficient space, you may not know how to regulate closeness and distance. If you grew up thinking that screaming and yelling is how people get their needs met, or that withdrawing and becoming isolated from others is how disagreements get settled, you were not taught a useful way of settling differences. If your childhood was replete with lies, deceit, rigid dictums, manipulation, neglect, mixed messages, intentional hurt, retaliation, betrayal, or physical or emotional abandonment, you likely came away from it with the wrong idea that people can't be trusted.

If fur was always flying in your home, it's easy to see why you might have technical difficulties with intimacy now. But there's another kind of early family dysfunction that occurs just as frequently and causes as much relational distress down the road. That's when parents deny their feelings or don't talk openly about them. When you grow up in a family that fights all the time, you at least know that expressing upset feelings is okay. But when you're raised in a household in which everything *seems* fine (except for the vague, subliminal tensions you just can't quite put your finger on), and you're constantly assured that everything is "just fine," it's harder to see what's missing. I bet you can guess what was lacking: the expression of emotions. Many families act as if it's legitimate to put everything on the table except what's going on inside them.

Perhaps you'd come home from school and find Mom crying in her bedroom, but when you'd ask what was wrong, she'd sniffle and say, "Nothing," or smile and insist, "I'm okay, really." Maybe the chill in the air from Mom and Dad giving each other the silent treatment for days on end was enough to make your home feel like an igloo, and it was nerve-racking trying to figure out exactly how bad things were between them. At least in a family in which emotions run high and are openly expressed, you know that people have and are allowed to show feelings. When you're raised in a home in which emotions seem not to exist, you start to question your own feelings — and everyone else's.

I hope you're starting to understand the myriad ways that your parents' lack of relationship skills may have been passed down to you. If you learned that getting attached to people would only make life worse, no wonder you'd choose cheesecake over a crony any day of the week. If you view relationships as iffy at best, and downright dangerous and scary at worst, it makes sense that you'd steer clear of them.

▄▀▄ Get Smart!

How did the way your parents related to you, each other, and other family members affect your ability to be in a healthy relationship now? How did their expression or nonexpression of emotions affect your relational skill set?

What Skills Do I Need to Learn in Order to Have Great Relationships?

Before I answer this question, take a moment to consider someone or several people you know who seem successful in developing and holding on to quality relationships. Maybe this role model is a distant relative, neighbor, coworker, or former teacher or coach. Think specifically about what makes you believe this individual excels at relationships. If you know several "stars" in this department, use them all to help you develop a mental checklist of qualities that help people relate well to others. This checklist will help you see that it's not essential to be outgoing, charming, charismatic, or smart in order to have positive, lasting relationships. In truth, relationship skills are not determined by whether your still waters run deep or you enjoy being the belle of the ball, by whether you have a GED or a PhD, or by whether you're well traveled or have never left your hometown. I guarantee that you have what it takes to develop and keep high-quality relationships. All you need to do is recognize what to look for in people that tells you they have reasonably good relational skills and some practice.

1. Look for People You Can Trust Emotionally

Trust is the basis of every relationship. If I get on an airplane, I trust that the pilot will know how to fly and land the plane. If I go to a dentist, I trust that he or she is competent to fill my cavities and adjust my bite correctly. I know that's not the kind of trust we think of when we talk about intimate relationships, but it has a strong bearing on the subject. What I'm saying is that we need to be able to trust people to represent themselves accurately.

When folks say they're kind and caring, it's vital for them to back it up with behavior that supports this statement. To trust people, we must know that who they think and say they are is reinforced by their actions.

Sometimes people tell us right off the bat that they're not good at long-term relationships, are scared of intimacy, aren't the marrying kind, or can't seem to get the hang of monogamy, and so on. We can usually trust that they're being honest, and we should feel grateful that they've given us fair warning about their relational deficits. But it's harder to spot people who aren't honest when they portray themselves in a loving, caring light. It's natural to want to trust that we won't have the wool pulled over our eyes, and that someone will continue to be our Prince or Princess Charming.

Learning how to trust is a skill. There are scores of ways you could have learned not to trust people in childhood, and I'm not going to describe them all here. If you don't trust people, you usually know it, to a greater or lesser extent, so let's start from the premise that you don't, and that you want to become skilled at trusting.

Start by noticing your gut impression when you initially meet someone. Simply observe the feeling that comes up, without judging or liking it. It can be especially difficult to make romantic connections when you're immediately attracted to someone and forget there's more to a relationship than physicality. So, along with noticing that someone is hot, observe his or her appearance and what message it's giving. Listen to how this person speaks — both the words and the tone — and pay attention to how he or she interacts with you and with others. Is this person kind and empathetic, or does he or she ridicule people with sarcasm or barely respond when others are speaking? Does this person love to tease people even when they don't seem to enjoy it? Although you're not purposely asking yourself if you can trust him or her — whether we're talking about a neighbor, coworker, or date — you're registering whether there's anything that would indicate this individual is not emotionally trustworthy.

Many people go wrong by trusting folks that everybody else finds untrustworthy. If your boss has a reputation for flirting with supervisees, even if he's been a perfect gentleman around you, you don't want to ignore the possibility that he will come on to you at some point. If the neighbors on your right and left tell you that the swell guy across the street has borrowed money from them and not returned it, tuck that nugget of information away, because it's an indication of his character. If your coworker gossips about everyone, it's not smart to trust her with your darkest secrets. Well, you get the idea.

You'll also want to be on top of your own issues, because we often take things personally and jump to (wrong) conclusions. For example, if you ask a new friend for help and she explains why she can't give it to you, don't immediately assume she's selfish and can't be counted on. If you have every reason to believe she's friendship material, you would be wise to give her another try. And this brings us to the most important way we gain information about people: by noticing their patterns of behavior. When I first moved to Sarasota, I met lots of people and put effort into making friends — going out of my way to speak with those who appeared to have potential and suggesting we make plans to get together. But I was careful to go slowly and wait long enough to see acquaintances over time before I made up my mind about how they fit into my life. Patterns take a while to develop, from weeks to months. People don't have to be perfect to make it onto my friend list, but they need to show a pattern of honesty, caring, and reciprocity before I would even consider counting them as intimates.

▞ Get Smart!

How trusting are you about personal matters? If you'd like to be more trusting, what holds you back? Fear of being hurt? Do you have a pattern of trusting too quickly, then getting disappointed?

2. Look for People Who Know How and When to Share about Their Personal Lives and Are Eager to Hear about Yours

I was once sitting in the lobby of an office building when the woman next to me struck up a conversation, giving me way more information than I could possibly want about her dysfunctional life. We all know people like that, who are only too happy to spill their guts indiscriminately. Alternatively, I've had acquaintances for years who barely said a word about their personal lives. They're always "fine," and when others discuss their own problems, these people go silent. Sometimes they ask a million questions about others, but never quite get around to sharing what's going on in their own little world. They may be great friendship material, but not for me. If I'm going to open up, it'll have to be even steven.

Once again, this is where patterns are important. I've met people who take a while to warm up, and it may take several interactions for them to slowly let me into their personal world. That's fine with me. If I see they're moving in that direction — if each time we meet they seem a bit more forthcoming — I'm game for hanging in there. I've had a few friends over the years who grew up in families where no one ever talked about their feelings, so they go really slowly when moving from acquaintanceship to intimacy, and I don't blame them. Just telling me that about their early upbringing is a trust-generating disclosure of vulnerability.

Many dysregulated eaters with dysfunctional childhoods have difficulty sharing. They fear they'll be rebuffed or ridiculed, or that their feelings will be a burden to others. When you feel this way, it's time to move out of memory and into the present and objectively gauge the other person in reality. Do they complain about you dumping your problems on them? Do they shut you and others off every time something personal is said? If someone cuts you off every time you share something intimate, that's different from telling you they can't always talk when you phone to ask for their advice on a personal matter.

The biggest relational difficulty I've observed in dysregulated eaters is that they often get into one-sided relationships in which they're the helpers and others are the helped. Of course, you don't want to be making mental tick marks when someone takes care of you or you take care of them. But you do want the feeling of mutuality and reciprocity. One of the worst positions you can put yourself in is being everyone's confidant. When you are, you have not only your problems but also theirs to contend with, and nowhere to vent. And once you're in that situation, how long do you think it will take before you're speeding toward a carbohydrate fix?

Get Smart!

How well balanced are your relationships in terms of sharing? Are you more often the helper than the helped because you feel less vulnerable and more powerful in that role? If you don't share when you need to, how does that affect your eating habits and your emotional stability?

3. Look for People Who Feel and Express Empathy

Clients often ask about the difference between sympathy and empathy. I explain it this way: with sympathy, someone feels bad *for* you; and with empathy, he or she feels bad *with* you. When something goes wrong, you want someone to validate what you are experiencing, which tells you that someone else has felt what you've felt or pretty darn close to it. For example, your friend may not have lost a child as you have, but he may have lost intimates that he loved deeply; and he can use those feelings to empathize with you.

Sympathy is fine as far as it goes, but when it comes to friendships, you really want someone who's able to slip on their hip boots and slog around in the muck with you. Another trait that is not empathy is what's called in clinical terms "parallel play." That's when you say that you just found out you may lose your job, and someone immediately shares their experience with having been laid off or fired. Usually they're trying to be helpful, and may eventually circle back to asking more about your situation and offering emotional validation and support. But sometimes they just continue on with their job-loss experience, and what you end up with is not a deep, emotional, satisfying connection but a recitation of your woes and a parallel recitation of theirs with little emotional exchange occurring.

This kind of dynamic is common in relationships and can be highly unsatisfying. You feel as if someone is in the ballpark with you — that is, on the same subject — but is not quite connecting with you. You may even sense that you've triggered something that makes it difficult for her to give you what you need — empathy. In these cases, the deficit is often not yours but hers. If someone isn't empathic and a good listener, she will never be the kind of friend you deserve.

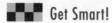 **Get Smart!**

Do people you're close to empathize with you, or do you wind up with sympathy or parallel play? How do you feel when someone empathizes with you? Why would you stay in a close relationship with someone who doesn't?

---

4. Look for People Who Have Good Boundaries

We first learn about boundaries through physical space. Your sister insists that you "stay out of my room!" Or your parents remind you not to leave your stuff in the common areas of the house. When you're raking leaves or shoveling snow, you learn pretty quickly where your neighbor's yard ends and yours begins. You come to recognize boundaries in school when you're told what you can and can't do on school property. Boundaries tell us: "this is my space" and "this is your space."

Of course, boundaries can be either rigid or flexible. If you're playing in a tennis tournament, you sure don't want to step over the line as you serve the ball. And there can be plenty of jurisdictional issues about where a crime has been committed, even if it's only a few yards over a state line. On the other hand, if you're sharing a dorm room, your things might accidentally end up on your roommate's side or his on yours, and you simply sort out what belongs to whom as you go along.

Boundaries regarding people are a bit more complex. Essentially, we're talking about folks knowing where their needs end and yours begin, and vice versa. Here are some examples of people who don't have good boundaries: A mother who tells her daughter, as I heard one say, "I'm cold. Put on a sweater." A father who blows up when you tell him that you decided not to attend his alma mater but wish to instead go to another college that is a better fit for you. A friend who steals your boyfriend. A coworker or boss who claims credit for a job well done — by you.

Some people simply think "what's yours is mine." They may also think "what's mine is yours," and maybe you can live with this and maybe you can't. But some people with poor boundaries really believe "what's yours is mine and what's mine is mine." As you notice, this leaves them with everything and you with nothing. This situation occurs when someone talks all about himself and doesn't let you get a word in edgewise. It arises when your roommate borrows your favorite purse but makes it clear you're to stay away from her stuff.

Boundary issues also surface when someone talks over you, eats your food without asking first if it's okay with you, copies your school or work ideas, and takes over a physical space that is yours. Needless to say, if someone touches you inappropriately, that's a mega boundary violation. Someone who wants to make all your decisions for you, or who always has to have things his way, is also exhibiting poor boundaries.

Two kinds of boundaries that portend relationship difficulties are those that are way too tight and those that are way too loose. Some people are inflexible; and when you're with them, things always have to be a certain way — their way. They need to drive and to pick the restaurant, won't share about a particular issue unless you've given your opinion first, and are generally pretty tightly wrapped in social settings. Other folks are loosey-goosey and have no clue that you're mortified when they share their sexual fantasies with your friends they've just met or flirt outrageously with your new boyfriend and then tell you later to stop being so uptight.

When assessing someone's boundaries, you'll pretty much want them to match yours. Sure, opposites attract, and someone with tight boundaries might get a kick out of someone who exhibits more flexibility, but these two personalities might not make it as best buds. Equally, if you're loud, and people at the other end of the bar can generally hear your every whisper, you might have difficulty being close friends with someone inclined to keep things to himself.

▰▰ Get Smart!

What kind of people are you drawn to, those with tight or loose boundaries? How have boundaries been a problem for you in relationships? How will you spot and avoid these problems in the future?

Although the skills I've just described will help you judge whether other people are relationship material, they also apply to you: are you trustworthy, empathic, willing to share and be vulnerable, and do you have reasonably good boundaries? More to the point for dysregulated eaters: do you set boundaries between yourself and others and hold people to them, or do you let others trample all over your borders and desires?

In my clinical experience, dysregulated eaters often don't have good boundaries or engage in relationships with people who do. It's more common for them to feel used and get stuck in a victim mentality, which leads to tremendous internal distress and an increased likelihood that they'll find solace in food.

You can't expect to connect with people who have good boundaries if you don't exhibit them yourself. Instead, you will likely find folks who have relationships *only* with those who have poor boundaries. Who else would put up with them?

Can't Expecting Too Much or Too Little of Relationships Drive Me to a Food Fix?

The answer, as you know too well, is that misplaced expectations certainly can trigger mindless eating. In a healthy partnership, the expectations of both parties are reasonable. Not all the time, of course, but most of the time. Work, romantic, and friendly relationships don't always start off with realistic expectations, but if both individuals are willing to talk about and work on improving their expectations, they can become a nonissue.

Say, for example, you are a teacher, and most of the teachers at your school work late and generally leave the building with a load of work to do at home. Naturally, the school principal is used to this and expects you, as the new teacher, to do the same. But if you became a teacher because you thought you'd get to leave school early and have time to play, well, I see storm clouds on the horizon. Or perhaps, because you're a terrific gourmet cook, your new housemates expect you to do most of the food prep, while you're thrilled to be living with three other people precisely because you're looking forward to the cooking being shared by all. Maybe you think that, because you've been dating the same woman for six months, the two of you are monogamous. That's the kind of subject you'd want to have a conversation about, not only because you don't want to get your heart broken but also because you don't want a sexually transmitted disease.

We all have conscious and unconscious expectations, and sometimes we don't even know we're expecting too little of a relationship. You may think the worst thing you can do is expect too much and be disappointed, but how about when you expect too little — and that's what you get? Either way, you're going to be disappointed! So often I hear clients describe not getting what they want from friends, lovers, spouses, bosses, parents, children, and coworkers, and it's because they've settled for so much less than they deserve. It's also crucial that you do not pick people you know can't give you what you want. Don't go into a relationship with the expectation that you can change a person who everyone, but you, can see has certain characteristics — ones that are clearly wrong for you (and maybe for anybody!).

One of the easiest skills to learn, in regard to expectations, is how to share them. Put your desires on the table and encourage the other person to do the same, whether that person is your supervisor, a budding friend, or your neighbor next door who seems to have more than a neighborly interest in you. It's fine to try to sense what someone wants, but there's nothing like having a heart-to-heart to make things perfectly clear.

Get Smart!

Do you go into relationships with your eyes wide open or tightly shut? Do you have realistic expectations in most relationships, or are you generally wearing rose-colored glasses? How comfortable are you when talking openly about what you expect and when asking other people about their expectations? Are you willing to speak openly in order to have better relationships?

What Other Relationship Skills Do I Need?

Which skills will keep your relationships in good working order, and keep *you* from eating your heart out? People who do well in relationships usually understand something about relational dynamics. For example, when people are stressed, in your experience, do they become upset and angry, or mellow? We all know exactly what happens, because we've experienced stress ourselves and recognize that the pressure can build up until we feel ready to explode. So try to understand the notion that, when your mother is preparing for a dinner party, she might not have time to check out your hot new shoes. Likewise, if someone lost his job last week, he might not want to hear that your boss is sending you to Paris next month to close a deal.

Also useful is your understanding that people often say things in the heat of the moment that they deeply regret, and usually feel awful about it, when they calm down. Don't get hung up on what someone said, but focus on her reaction when you explain how hurt you felt. Watch for patterns. If someone is defensive and often blows up at you, stay away — even if she apologizes profusely every time. To lean heavily on a few clichés, apologies are a dime a dozen, but someone who changes his behavior at your request is putting his money where his mouth is and is worth his weight in gold.

Remember, too, that what comes out of someone's mouth, even if it has your name attached to it, is always about the person speaking. It comes from *their* brain, *their* perception, and *their* viewpoint. This means it's not necessarily true. As one person said on my Food and Feelings message board, "Just because someone says you're a car, do you sleep in the garage?" People can say all sorts of things about you, and every word may be untrue. The better you know yourself, and the more honestly you can identify your strengths and weaknesses, the better you'll recognize when what people say about you is spot on, or when they're just blowing smoke through their hats to make themselves feel better. I assure you, there's a great deal of that going around.

Here's a psychologically oriented skill that will help you weather relationships: recognizing that people often say rotten things about you that are true of themselves. This process is called *projection* and is triggered by a person's discomfort about a trait they have — say, they can be unnecessarily sarcastic. They may accuse you, the least derisive person in the universe, of mocking others. Don't buy into it if it's not who you know yourself to be, no matter how much they insist. Understand that they're simply uncomfortable with who they are and will use this defense mechanism often to feel more comfortable about themselves.

Also remember that there are many Very Difficult People (VDPs) in this world. They are everywhere and, over time, are easily identifiable if you know how to spot them. In most cases, they're difficult for everyone, but not always. Sometimes their positive traits are so overwhelmingly lovable that you might put up with their negative ones. Say you know someone who can be counted on to make you laugh, someone who can't help looking on the bright side of life, but who always needs to be right. A person who can't stand being wrong is generally difficult to be around, but you may choose to tolerate this particular friend because of her upbeat, fun-loving nature.

Another kind of VDP may be your boss who is nitpicky and critical: no one wants to work for him when you're on vacation. The pleasing part of him is that if someone says anything bad about you, he'll go to bat for you every time. He's as loyal as your dog, Rover, and you can't say that about everyone. You know how difficult he can be, but you tolerate working for him because you also know he's got your back.

Then again, how about your next-door neighbor who's standoffish? The rest of the block thinks he's a cold fish, but he was the only one on the block to shovel your driveway when you were bedridden with pneumonia. You can barely get a wave out of him in the morning when you both head off to work, but there he was, knee deep in snow, digging out your car just in case you were feeling better and needed it, when all your so-called friendly neighbors were drinking hot cocoa inside their toasty kitchens.

My point is that people are complicated and so are relationships. Just because you have excellent skills in building and maintaining relationships doesn't mean they'll run smoothly or that things won't go awry. One thing I can promise you is that, even in the best of relationships, you will at times feel hurt, angry, taken aback, frustrated, and disappointed. In a healthy relationship, you won't feel these emotions often, and when you do you'll be able to talk through your feelings with the other person and usually come away feeling better about yourself and even the relationship. The fact is that a thorough airing of grievances can go a long way toward strengthening a relationship and making two people feel closer. All relationships have their ups and downs; that's the nature of the beast.

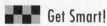 ## Get Smart!

Do you take what others say too personally or gloss over hurts that occur repeatedly? Are you attracted to VDPs in the hopes of changing them? How astute are you at spotting and handling VDPs?

Skill Boosters

1. Make a list of the reasons that food is not your friend. Make a list of the reasons that friendship is better than nonhunger eating.

2. List the qualities you would like in a friend, boss, coworker, date, and mate.

3. What did your parents tell you about trust in relationships growing up?

4. What behaviors or attitudes did your parents model with each other that gave you a positive or negative impression of relationships?

5. Reflect on what your own experiences with relationships have taught you, especially the part you played in creating negative experiences.

6. Notice the qualities of people with whom you're in relationships, and identify which qualities improve connection and which ones detract from it.

7. Share your expectations with a boss, date, friend, neighbor, or coworker and ask them to share their expectations of the relationship with you.

8. Identify the VDPs in your life, what makes them so difficult, and how you will handle them, which may include letting them go from your life.

9. Make a point of noting when people are projecting, which means blaming you for a quality you may or may not have but they certainly do.
10. How could you improve yourself and become a better partner in any relationship?

In chapter 6, you'll learn how to avoid going to extremes, to keep yourself pleasantly centered and balanced in terms of emotions, activities, and boundaries with others.

CHAPTER 6

Self-Regulation

There's Something Besides an On-Off Switch?

Self-regulation is not a term we hear often in everyday life, but it's exactly what's not happening when people have difficulty managing eating and other behaviors. If you're a dysregulated eater you may find that you have trouble knowing when enough is enough in other areas of life as well. You may overwork or underexercise, overdo taking care of friends and neglect your self-care, or spend an inordinate amount of time piddling around and too little getting major tasks done.

Of course, biology and genetics play a huge role in our relationship to food and perhaps, as well, in our ability to regulate other activities. I suspect there's a biological component to many of our proclivities, one that we'll uncover one day, just as science has discovered that the trait of sensitivity (as in, "Oh, you're just too sensitive") may have an underlying biochemical basis for some individuals. But, biology aside, being able to self-regulate is an essential skill that, when done effectively, will make your whole life far more manageable and enjoyable.

At the heart of the self-regulation conflict is a yearning for, and yo-yoing back and forth between, structure and freedom. You know how it is when you have a wild feeding frenzy and the next day vow to go on a diet, or you lounge around the house all day as you shamefully, guiltily, give in to inertia, then get with the program and work far into the night to finish your chores. Think of it this way: When you become sufficiently uncomfortable with having no rules for eating, you think that imposing many rules is the answer and you begin your new diet. When you avoid your chores for long enough, you berate yourself for being a lazy head and, in a panic, barrel through everything on your to-do list until you're ready to drop. Alternatively, you get into a routine like going to the gym or cleaning up after yourself daily until you're sick of it, then you drop it completely. The problem is that you enjoy or value routine for only a short while, until it starts to feel like pressure — or prison — and then you long to break away and be footloose and fancy-free once more.

I hope you recognize that self-regulation is, in part, about acknowledging and respecting your need — or, rather, the very human need — for both freedom *and* structure. One is not good and the other bad; one is not better than the other. Both, in fact, are value neutral. You require some of each to lead a balanced and satisfying life.

This may be a brand-new, shocking — and, perhaps even disturbing — concept to you. Rather than hurl yourself from structure to freedom and back again, knowing you'll never stop pinging and ponging if you keep it up, consider how you might move from freedom to a teensy bit more structure, or from structure to a tad more loosening up. No need to go whole hog in either direction. Better to avoid both extremes of dysregulation and simply pay attention to sensing your need for more structure or freedom. In this case, having a little of each goes a long way toward keeping you in balance.

Get Smart!

How do you feel when your routines become too rigid or excessive? How do you feel when you don't have or don't follow routines at all? Specifically, what could you do to remain more in balance?

Now, back to the term *self-regulation*. If you're not exactly sure what I mean by it, try these examples on for size:

- You hardly ever exercise, but you sporadically go on intense weekend boot camps, which, the next day, make your body feel as if it's been run over by a truck.
- When you join a gym, you insist on going either every day or for two hours at a clip, even though neither is feasible given your schedule, so you eventually stop going altogether.
- You rarely buy clothes for yourself, but when you do it's a mega shopping spree and you come home with oodles of items that you look at and think, "When will I ever wear this?"
- You have a hard time leaving work on time almost every night, even though pretty much everyone else zips out the door at five sharp.
- Your home is either a mess or spotless.
- You usually let other people make decisions for you, which builds up a head of resentment in you until, one day, you put your foot down and freak out everyone when you insist, irrationally, that some petty thing must be done your way.
- You spend so much time with your social network in cyberspace that you miss out on real time with friends, so you unsubscribe to all your favorite sites, until you're in such deep withdrawal that you sign up again on them all.
- You either stuff your feelings or can't stop crying, screaming, or moping around.
- You pledge to go to sleep at a reasonable hour and do it self-righteously for a week, then lapse back into hitting the sack long after your body and mind have quit for the day.
- If you can't do something perfectly, or at least exceedingly well, you either don't do it at all or you're miserable the whole time you're doing it, because you feel like a failure.

These may seem like normal, everyday actions to you, but they're examples of dysregulation. It's as if you were born with only an on-off switch and no calibration in between. If you have dimmer switches on the lights in your home, you know what I mean by what's "in between": there's a whole range between blindingly bright light and dim light in which you can barely see your hand. Just as the volume control on your iPhone or TV is a continuum, you, as a human instrument, also possess a finely tuned control mechanism, but one that's been stuck in the on-off position. The skill you want to develop is to identify, value, and use its calibrations.

 Get Smart!

Do any of the examples here ring true? As you consider activities other than eating, do you think you might have more general problems with effectively regulating yourself, other than around food?

How wonderful would it be for you to feel nuances of hunger, to not simply feel famished or stuffed but to feel all the stops along the way — not quite hungry, mildly hungry, almost full, and so on? Can you imagine how satisfying it would be to know that you'll recognize and accept when a job is finished, even if it's not done perfectly? Can you imagine listening to your body so that you'll give it just the right amount of sleep, exercise, rest, and stimulation most of the time?

By acquiring both physical and emotional self-regulation skills, you'll learn to do all that and more. In order for this to happen, however, you'll need to deeply connect to your body. I don't mean connect in the way too many dysregulated eaters connect to their bodies by judging and obsessing about their size or appearance. I mean being aware of your internal shifts in physical sensation and noticing what you feel when your body is in different states.

Here are examples of dysregulated and regulated responses. When your dysregulated self is hiking with friends, you notice that you're sadly out of shape and not keeping up, that you're huffing and puffing your way along. Every time you fall behind, you admonish yourself to catch up. You pretend you don't feel tired, and you override your muscles' screams for you to slow down or stop and rest. Rather than speak up and ask your friends to sit down for a bit and enjoy the scenery, you stay mum until your calves are burning and you're so winded you can barely speak. When you've recovered enough breath, you angrily wheeze out your belief that your friends don't care about you or they would have walked more slowly, and you announce that you're giving up and going home.

A version of yourself more skilled at self-regulation might approach this outing as follows. First off, rather than impulsively agree to the hike, you'd think long and hard beforehand about whether you'll be able to keep up with your friends, based on how fit you are compared to them. You wouldn't let shame prevent you from telling your friends ahead of time that you just might need to go a little slower than everyone else, and you would ask whether that would be okay with the group. Then you'd try to do a bit more walking or other exercise every day before the hike in order to build up some stamina, and during the hike you would go at a pace comfortable for you. You'd pay serious attention to what your body was telling you every inch of the way and even mention to your friends how you were doing so they could take your pace into account.

Can you see the difference in these examples — how you're monitoring yourself appropriately or not? I use this situation to illustrate that regulation involves more than an on-off switch, and how keenly tuned into our bodies we must be to pace ourselves effectively in any kind of activity. Moreover, there's an emotional component going on here as well. In the first instance, you're ashamed and, therefore, silent until you abruptly blow up and give up. In the second, you nonjudgmentally stay in touch with what you're feeling along the way and are comfortable sharing with others. The hike becomes not an all-or-nothing challenge but an enjoyable, satisfying physical and social activity.

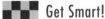 **Get Smart!**

Do you tend to make all-or-nothing choices and see only perfection or failure? Do you often override what your body and emotions are telling you and habitually either underdo or overdo?

How Can I Learn to Better Self-Regulate?

Try this exercise. Get up and stand near something you can hold on to, like a table or the back of a chair. Now lift one foot slightly off the ground and let go of whatever you're holding on to. Observe how your body shifts a teensy bit in one direction, then the other, to stay balanced. Okay, end of exercise. Notice how naturally you shifted your body. You didn't let yourself fall down, then get up. Your mind and body made quick, automatic observations and adjustments to maintain balance.

The skill of self-regulation requires this kind of monitoring and correction. In fact, in many ways, you already do it every day. When you're cooking and the pan gets too hot, you adjust the temperature. You don't switch it off completely, do you? Ditto when the shower water threatens to either scald or freeze you. Similarly, you shift your body around on a crowded bus or subway so that you have enough space for yourself, but you also make room for others. You may not think of these behaviors as self-regulation, but they are.

The key is to stay connected to what you're thinking and feeling physically and emotionally at all times, except when you wish to intentionally go unconscious in a healthy way (for more about living consciously, see chapter 4). To become skilled at self-regulation, you also want to frequently ask yourself if you are getting or doing too much or too little. Eventually you will sense enoughness; but to learn how this sense of sufficiency is experienced in your mind and body, you will first have to pay exquisite attention.

In fact, right now, ask yourself these questions: Am I tired of reading this chapter or eager to continue learning more? Am I tired of this book or eager to read on? Am I hungry, and if so, am I hungry enough to eat? How is my body feeling — does it want to stay in the position it's resting in or move around a bit?

What you're doing is scanning yourself to identify what's going on inside you. For now, it's important to stop whatever you're doing when you're scanning, but when you get better at it, you'll be able to do it semi-consciously — although you'll still probably want to pause at times to get a better read on exactly what you're feeling. For example, as I'm typing away, I'm noticing that I'm slightly hungry as it approaches the noon hour, when I usually break for lunch. I don't have to do anything with this information right now except to note it. The next time I notice, my hunger will likely be stronger, and at some point it will tell me to get up and eat! This skill kicked in last night as well, when I was trying my darndest to finish a chapter and was getting more and more fatigued. Finally, my body gave me the signal to go to bed and I did, knowing that in the morning I'd pick up writing where I left off. That's how self-regulation works.

A warning about the one thing you don't want to do to enhance your sense of regulation, and which, unfortunately, I suspect is a method for determining enoughness that you've been using far too long: being guided by what others say is enough for you. This dynamic generally begins in childhood when you're habitually discouraged from sensing what's enough for yourself. When you're told by others what you feel or should feel or how much or how little you should have or do, you don't develop the ability to decide for yourself. Sadly, when parents refuse to validate the idea that only you know what's enough for yourself (age appropriately, of course) and you end up following their guidelines rather than your own, you start to lose your ability to sense sufficiency.

For example, let's say that as a child you used to love drawing and could do it for hours. Sure, you would have to stop once in a while for food, sleep, school, socializing, exercise, homework, and spending time with the family. If your parents were both jocks, they might have told you that you were spending too much time drawing and that this was bad for you. Or they even might have taken away your drawing materials because you wouldn't give them up voluntarily. Their actions could certainly have given you the impression that you didn't have a good sense of what was enough or too much for you. Of course, your parents may have simply wanted you to be a well-rounded child, but that doesn't mean this is the message you received. What you may have internalized is that, left to your own devices, you didn't know when enough was enough. When parents occasionally guide us toward enoughness, it doesn't become an issue. When they do it too often, we stop trying to sense adequacy within ourselves.

Alternatively, maybe you had parents who thought you had talent at the piano (perhaps you even did) and made you practice for hours on end when you hated it. Let's say that every time you tried to get out of practicing, you were told you weren't doing enough to be successful — when you didn't care a fig if you ever played "Chopsticks" again. You probably didn't understand that your parents wanted you to use your talent, and instead you internalized the message that you didn't know what was enough for yourself. Again, if on occasion they forced you to do certain activities against your will, that's okay. But if they frequently imposed their will on you and overrode your natural inclinations, you might have come to believe that others know better than you do when enough is enough.

In both of these examples, I'm not parent bashing. I'm trying to show you how subtle messages about enoughness creep into us in childhood. What if everyone is doing more of something and you want to do less? What if everyone is doing less and you want to do more? When you were growing up, were you, for the most part, encouraged to make your own decisions regardless of others' preferences, or was only homogeneity and conformity acceptable in your family? Could you eat as much or as little as you wanted most of the time, or was there a set portion you were given, which may have left you hungry or stuffed, that you had to eat — and never mind trying to change your parents' minds?

On the other hand, maybe your parents showed little interest in helping you figure out what was the right amount of anything for you, so that you were always struggling with what was too much or too little. For instance, maybe you tried so hard to do things that were way above your academic level that you ended up feeling like a failure. A little explanation from your parents about overreaching would have come in handy right there. Or perhaps you needed a little push to try harder to make friends when you moved to a new school, and you never received it from your parents so you gave up and simply spent all your time alone in your room. Had you been encouraged a bit, that might have been just enough of a nudge to help you become more sociable in an unfamiliar environment.

▰▰ Get Smart!

How did your parents influence your ability to self-regulate when you were a child? Were you regularly coerced into doing or taking too much or too little? Were you allowed, at the appropriate age, to make decisions about what was enough for yourself? What kind of role models were your parents in the self-regulation department? What effect does their past modeling in your childhood have on your self-regulation today?

If Nobody Taught Me to Figure Out What's Enough, How Will I Ever Know?

I've written before about what I believe many dysregulated eaters suffer from, which I call an "enough" disorder. Good thing it's treatable. So, let's get started. First off, make a list of the areas in which you don't know when enough is enough — that is, areas in which you're not sure what amount is too little, just right, or too much. Here are some possibilities: food, sleep, rest, self-care, weight, work, play, child care, exercise, medical attention, taking medication, helping friends, and carving out time for yourself. To start practicing identifying nuance, note whether you have a lot of difficulty in an area or just a little. After all, I'm sure you're better at sensing sufficiency in some areas than in others.

Now, take one particular area in which you already do fairly well, and see if you can tweak it to improve. Let's say you usually get enough sleep, but not on vacation, when you just want to stay up and have a good time — something that doesn't work so well when you awaken in the morning bleary-eyed with a full day of activity planned. How could you arrange for a better balance of sleep and wakefulness when you're on vacation? Do you need to reduce your fear of missing out on fun, or pace yourself better during the day? Maybe you could take a brief nap during the afternoon to be able to stay up later. Or maybe you could restructure your vacation so that you wouldn't be trying to cram so many activities into each day.

When you're done with that, take a more difficult area — say, making sure that you take enough time for yourself and don't lavish it all on family members. Consider how you feel about caring for yourself, especially if it causes you to feel selfish and guilty. Explore where that wrongheaded conviction comes from, and counter it with a belief like: "It's not selfish to take care of myself" or "I need to take care of myself so I can take care of others." Then make a plan to start doing less for your family and more for yourself. Maybe the kids will get to make dinner one night a week, and maybe you'll buy takeout another night so that you have time to relax after a hard day's work. Perhaps they can ride their bikes rather than expect you to shuttle them in the car to all their activities, or they can carpool with other kids. Think hard: how can I carve out important time for myself, even if I only sit in my room and stare at my navel?

I hope you're getting the idea of how to develop the skill of knowing what's enough, which is another way of saying: what is exactly right for you. Remember Goldilocks and the porridge that was "not too hot and not too cold," and the bed that was "not too little and not too big but just right"? That's what you're trying to determine — what feels just right to you. Sufficiency is a felt sense, a sensation that hits you in your gut when you know you have reached it. Until then, a little voice in your head whispers, "Okay, you can do [or have] a little more." And when you get to "just right," that voice gets louder and insists, "There, stop there, that's precisely right." Consider when you've had that feeling — with food, time at the beach, completing a work project, decorating your house, playing tennis, hanging with friends, or working in the garden. If you listen closely, you will almost always know when enough is enough. Conversely, you can be sure that if you don't pay attention to it, you will soon hear another voice insisting, "You did it again — too much, too much!"

The good news is that as you get better at tuning into sufficiency in one area, this proficiency will spread throughout other areas. Some examples:

- When you regularly stop eating at the point when you reach satiation, you may start to realize you've had it with friends who go on and on about their problems and don't leave any time for you to talk about your life. Then you might nicely let them know that you have some things you'd like to share before a call ends, or you may even cut them off and tell them you have to go because you have things to do.

- You might be doing so many activities to benefit your community that you have little time to spend with your own family. In that case, you might try cutting back your hours as a volunteer at the women's shelter gift shop. If you still don't have enough family time, maybe you'll let your term as president of the PTA run out and not seek that office again. Soon you'll recognize that doing too much of anything doesn't feel right, and you'll become better attuned to being in balance.

- If you've been a jock, you might notice that you're no longer seriously interested in competitive skiing or tennis but are really looking to enjoy yourself socially, get a good workout, and engage in these sports at a less taxing level. As you pressure yourself less in athletic prowess, you might realize how hard you've pushed yourself in most areas and decide to take it a little easier in life, period.

■■■ Get Smart!

What beliefs would you like to change in order to encourage yourself to sense when you're "just fine"? Pay particular attention to unhealthy beliefs about not deserving much, about needing to give more to others than to yourself, and about self-care equaling selfishness. How do you feel about learning to identify enoughness — excited, a little nervous, a mix of both?

So Is That It on the Self-Regulation Front?

Well, not exactly. Not only do you want to move away from all-or-nothing thinking, as well as from underdoing and overdoing certain behaviors, but you also want to develop skills that enable you to reregulate yourself fairly easily when you become emotionally dysregulated (as we all do at times).

Emotional dysregulation is something you're all too familiar with, although you may never have called it that. To comprehend the term, you first have to understand what it means to be emotionally regulated. In that state, you might say you're on an even keel, in stasis. Either nothing in particular is distressing you, or you might notice that you're a tad miffed at your spouse or anxious about an upcoming evaluation by your boss. Either way, the feeling isn't strong enough to upset or threaten your equilibrium and inner peace. Emotion isn't spilling over and making your heart beat like a drum, or making your thoughts flit around inside your head like bats in a cave.

Dysregulation happens when your nervous system responds as if you're under attack, when you suddenly feel as if you're losing centeredness or control of your emotions. You're intensely aware of a powerful affect, and you sense a strong need for action — that is, a need to do or say something to feel better. Dysregulation can happen when you recall something that upsets you (remember our discussion of memory triggers in chapter 3) — you think back to finding pot in your daughter's makeup case this morning when you were searching for the lipstick she borrowed from you; or you are nagged by the recollection of that horrible argument you had with your college roommate when she came to visit for the weekend, and how she stormed out the door without saying good-bye; or you remember that it's the one-year anniversary of your father's death and feel grief-stricken.

Because your memory is chock-full of events that could upset (or dysregulate) you, all you need to do is light upon one of them and, wham, you're flooded with unwanted affect. Your life at the moment may actually be fine and dandy; but according to the miscue you received internally, you believe it isn't, and you're off and running. For us to become dysregulated, we don't need "bad" things to happen externally. We can cause dysregulation all by our little old selves!

But, life being what it is (unpredictable, not arranged for our comfort or convenience), events from the environment do influence us and can easily cause dysregulation: Your son's principal may call to say little Freddy got into a fight and has a bloody nose. Your boss might toss a proposal on your desk at 4:40 that needs to be proofread posthaste, not caring (or even knowing) that you have to pick up your mother from the hairdresser's at 5:00 sharp. Or it's your birthday, and your best friend may cancel dinner plans at the last minute because she has the stomach flu and is heading home for the night, leaving you with an empty evening ahead.

Both recall-triggered and externally generated events can powerfully dysregulate us emotionally. There we are, tooling along thinking all is right with the world, and suddenly we're plunging down the rabbit hole like Alice. It may literally feel as if one moment we're fine and the next we're not. Suddenly you recall something upsetting and can't imagine how you'd forgotten it for even a minute, or an external event slams into you and knocks the wind out of you. Either way, if you don't have the skills to reregulate yourself quickly, you're going to be in a pickle.

Is There Truly a Better Reregulator Than Food?

There had better be, hadn't there? Or you've wasted your money on this book. Of course there are better ways to reregulate yourself than eating. One question I ask clients is: What would you do to feel better if there were no such thing as food in the world? That is, what if it had never existed, and you'd never heard of such a thing? Please don't answer that you wouldn't do *anything* if food weren't around. There *is* something called self-preservation, which would propel you to find a way back to equilibrium. Maybe it wouldn't be a healthy activity; you might choose alcohol or drugs. Or perhaps you would do something only marginally healthy, like throw yourself into work even though you're exhausted, or call all your friends even though it's the middle of the night. My point is that you would find *something* to help you regroup, rather than suffer ongoing dysregulation.

I am intentionally not listing all the ways that you can bring emotions back into stasis. Some techniques can be found in chapter 3. Others can be found in my *Food and Feelings Workbook*. You may already know ways to comfort yourself, and you may either practice them sporadically or wish you did even that much. There is no magic way to reestablish stasis, and people who are skilled in doing so recognize that fact. Sometimes you just have to wait for an intense feeling to pass like a storm, knowing that you will feel peace once again when it's spent. Other times you'll want to take quick action so that the intensity of the emotion doesn't escalate.

One of the worst things you can tell yourself is how awful you feel or how terrible the event you're reacting to is. The goal is to minimize the threat of whatever is upsetting you — by talking to yourself or distracting yourself with an activity that will draw your attention away from your inner turmoil. Think self-soothe, self-soothe, self-soothe. And you'll notice that, eventually, the cortisol level in your body will drop, along with your heart rate, and you'll feel calmer.

Sometimes you can will yourself to calm down by acknowledging that you're dysregulated. I actually remind myself that this is what's going on in me and instruct myself to reregulate myself. This statement points my mind and body in the right direction and helps move me toward tranquility.

It also puts some distance between my perception of what's going on and what really is happening. Recognizing dysregulation is key to knowing what to do with it. You're not crazy, the world isn't going to end, and life as we know it isn't going to be extinguished. You may feel crazy inside, but when you give that sensation a name — dysregulation — then you have a chance to think clearly about your options, which are based on avoiding doing or saying anything to increase your distress, and doing and saying everything healthy you can think of to decrease it.

▰▰ Get Smart!

How do you feel about the term *dysregulation?* What are your own physical and mental signs of dysregulation? What are the most effective ways, not involving food, that you've found to reregulate yourself? Which ones might you try that you don't do now?

Can I Prevent Dysregulation?

You can prevent or avoid some, but not all, dysregulation. For example, what if you know that every time you visit Grandma, who barely knows you now, and whose dementia has turned her into a confused recluse, you leave distressed and drive through the Dairy Queen to console yourself? You now understand that visiting her dysregulates your nervous system, and your upset sometimes leaches into the rest of the day. You could certainly decide to stop visiting her, but that might make you feel bad and wouldn't be fair to Grandma.

What can you do to stop yourself from feeling so upset while you're with her? You can bring a magazine to leaf through while Grandma is resting her eyes, read to her, accept that her confusion and inability to recognize you is natural, take a break during the visit to call a friend, play some music your grandmother and you can enjoy together, do deep breathing exercises, or plan an enjoyable activity that you will do right after the visit. You can remind yourself that you'll sort out all your feelings when you get home — without food as a companion. These are some, certainly not all, of the things you can do to prevent yourself from careening over an emotional cliff.

And if you're able to contain your distress fairly well, you just may be able to get it back down to zero more quickly. Let's face it, we don't think rationally when we're upset; when we're in distress, our only drive is to reduce emotional discomfort posthaste. If you end your visit to Grandma in a clearer, more tranquil state of mind — in other words, if your distress level isn't rocketing off the charts — it's more likely that you'll make the wiser choice to circumvent the Dairy Queen.

You can also prevent dysregulation by avoiding unhappy memories and not triggering upset feelings. If thinking about the money you're losing on the cruise you had to cancel owing to acute appendicitis keeps making your blood boil — need I say it? — don't continue to retrieve and replay that recollection. Remind yourself that there's nothing you can do, and that you're only ruining the pleasant present by revisiting that memory. Would you keep rewatching a movie that upset you? Of course not. Well, treat memories the same way.

People who easily become dysregulated tend to assume that all instances of distress are of equal value, when they certainly are not. One comforting strategy is to remind yourself that some things are worth getting into a lather over, and some things simply are not. Temporarily losing your phone service, for example, is likely to affect you more than having your cable TV service go on the fritz. It's not a necessity to watch TV, but you might be waiting for an important business or personal call.

Moreover, people skilled in self-regulation generally try to avoid Very Difficult People (remember the VDPs from chapter 5?), who can be exceedingly dysregulating to be around. If you have the option to do so, choose not to hang around VDPs, who often lack appropriate interpersonal skills and boundaries. In fact, many VDPs are highly dysregulated themselves or cause others to be. Skilled self-regulators go out of their way to avoid VDPs as friends, and in social or work situations they try to minimize contact with them. If the chair of your condo board is a pain in the butt, you might have to put up with him during your monthly meetings, but you surely don't have to go out for a drink with him or have him and his wife over for dinner. If your doctor's nurse is an argumentative

person with a lousy disposition, recognize this fact, don't take it personally, and make sure to avoid getting into a discussion with her about anything except your specific medical matters.

Now, I bet you're thinking, "Well, what about family? What's she
going to do, tell me to never see my family again?" In some cases, absolutely, but not in most cases. How wonderful that we live in a huge nation,
and in a world with so many countries and continents. The fact is, in most
instances, we don't need to live near family. We may wrongly believe that
it's our duty, and may feel guilty as hell if we don't choose to reside near
them, but it is almost always a choice.

Frankly, some family members are just too abusive to be around, and
you have every right to choose not to spend time with them. But if you're
thinking of estranging yourself from family, it's a good idea to first talk
about it with someone you trust, and perhaps even with a professional.
This is a big step for most people who undertake it. But when family members dysregulate you so much that it's difficult for you to live the functional life you want and deserve, you may need to keep your distance — at
least for now. This also means no phone calls, emails, and texts.

Many people don't need to escape their families but do need to pro-
ceed with caution around them. Knowing that your family has the ability
to dysregulate you is helpful, and so are all the techniques for minimizing
upset feelings and reregulating yourself as quickly and deftly as possible. There's a skill you can practice called maintaining "caring distance,"
which is exactly that: giving family members some of what they need and
only what you can give in a detached way. This is an excellent strategy for
avoiding doing either too much or too little with them. The goal is to try
to do right by them and by yourself without much emotional intensity.

For example, when nurses' aides change the underwear of inconti-
nent people, they do it without a great deal of emotional attachment to
their charges; they see the task as part of the job. You can think of caring
for people you don't much like in this same way. You can do your duty
without having intimate feelings for them. People who are skilled at self-
regulation use this approach in order to stay regulated while doing what
they feel is necessary to keep their own self-respect and integrity — and
sanity.

One more word about how people become dysregulated: it happens when they don't take care of business and, therefore, end up creating a crisis for themselves. If you wait until the last minute to pay your taxes, you're going to feel frazzled on April 14. If you keep putting off a tooth extraction in order to avoid the pain of surgery, then the more pain your tooth gives you, the more emotionally distressed you're going to feel. If you grew up in a household in which there were frequent crises — Mom's tantrums, Dad's unemployment, evictions, or parental separations — crises may be what you're familiar with, which is why you continue to generate them to this day.

If so, talking to a professional will help you understand the roots of this pattern, and you can learn how to bring it to an end. Just because you grew up on a roller coaster doesn't mean you want to continue riding it. You'll be amazed at how reducing the number of crises in your life helps you stay regulated.

▦ Get Smart!

Is there anyone you need to maintain a caring distance from? How will doing so help you prevent emotional dysregulation? What can you do to avoid spending time locked into memories of disturbing events that distress you? Make a list of VDPs you want to steer clear of, and another list of those you want to minimize contact with whenever possible.

Trust me, you'll feel so much better when you're more adept at self-regulation. I don't mean you'll simply be happier with how you handle food; you'll also find yourself more relaxed. You'll feel more competent to face the world and confident in your ability to handle whatever crisis comes along. You don't have to be perfect at maintaining your equilibrium, but you do want to feel skilled at it. It will take time and practice — and numerous failures that you'll learn from — so don't expect success right away. Learn from each mistake, and make note of what keeps you regulated and returns you rapidly back to stasis when you become dysregulated.

Skill Boosters

1. Make a list of the behaviors you wish to regulate — for example, your behaviors around food, at work, while parenting, while doing more for yourself and less for others, and so on.

2. Notice things that exist on a continuum: volume controls, traffic that slows down and speeds up slowly, music that fades or grows louder, waning sunsets, and so on. This will help you recognize that most of life is measured in increments.

3. Ask yourself how you're feeling at the moment, to see if you're slowly starting to dysregulate, and then do something to nip the process in the bud.

4. Rather than hold in your feelings or opinions until you're like a balloon ready to burst, let feelings out little by little until you're fairly well deflated.

5. Examine your beliefs about success, perfection, and failure and change the ones that drive you to extremes.

6. Make a point of leaving some tasks unfinished, or done imperfectly, every once in a while.

7. At least a few times a day, scan your feelings and focus on whether you're approaching satisfaction or adequacy.

8. Practice stopping eating as soon as you're no longer hungry (you'll be surprised at how little food you need to actually quell hunger).

9. Find some humor in having an enoughness disorder, instead of being ashamed of or frustrated with it.

10. If getting to bed on time is a problem, check in with yourself every fifteen minutes and, without judging or fighting it, rate your tiredness level.

11. Stop looking to others to tell you what's enough for you, and look inward instead.

12. Make a list of the physical and mental signals that indicate you're becoming emotionally dysregulated.

13. Notice when you get bored with, or tired while doing, an activity and how much longer you continue with it beyond what is satisfying or sufficient.

14. Observe when people become dysregulated around you, and the physical and emotional changes that occur in them.
15. Make a list of VDPs in your family, circle of friends and acquaintances, workplace, and community, and decide how you're going to stay regulated around them.

In chapter 7, you'll learn how to think rationally, lucidly, and to make evidence-based decisions that are in your best interest.

CHAPTER 7

Problem Solving and Critical Thinking

Is Critical Thinking Different from Thinking Critically about Myself?

Much of our view of life is shaped by how we look at what we call problems. Many people see problems as pesky annoyances that keep getting in the way of permanent happiness and success — like debris on the garden path. They believe that if they could only solve all their problems, life would be grand and they could simply kick back and enjoy themselves to the end of their days. Ah, what a world that would be. But, alas, it is not the one in which we live. Instead, our world is filled with large and small problems galore, so we might as well give up the dream that they'll disappear, and learn how to live with them.

You know what I mean — if it's not the washing machine breaking down, it's baby Alice getting an ear infection, or the new boss turning out to be a tyrant, or rabbits demolishing your first vegetable garden. I could go on, but I'm sure you are entirely familiar with what I mean. Problems are like weeds: as soon as one is vanquished, another pops up — at least that's the way it seems.

And this sense of "how it *seems*" is what holds the key to unlocking one problem with problems. How often do you notice what goes wrong, but not what goes right? Many dysregulated eaters tend to look only at the negatives and disregard the positives, so much so that I often start my therapy or coaching sessions by saying, "So, tell me what's going on in your life that's positive, and a change for the better, since we last talked." For some clients that's really a showstopper!

Here's why my question about change is necessary, and how a conversation would go if I didn't instruct clients to share the bright side of their lives. I'd inevitably hear, "Well, I had the flu all week, and since I was home a lot with nothing to do, and was feeling sorry for myself, I noshed my way through the day when I really didn't even feel like eating, since I was so sick." My client would go on to tell me in excruciating detail every "bad" food she ate or overate and how frustrated she is with herself, complaining the entire session about her food failures, if I let her. Then, at the tail end of our conversation, she'd add, "Oh, and my husband and I started couples counseling, which went great. He was so into talking about improving our marriage that I cried right there in the therapist's office, and things have been really good between us since then."

The fact that this client had taken this gigantic step in a courageous, life-changing direction would have nearly slipped through the cracks. In her mind, how could it possibly take precedence over the mindless eating she'd been doing? This is often the way a dysregulated eater thinks, and I wouldn't be surprised if you do, too. I understand that when you speak with a therapist, you automatically cough up the things going wrong in your life — after all, isn't that the purpose of a therapist, to fix your problems? — but I don't believe this is all that's going on. In my experience, dysregulated eaters tend to evaluate their days, weeks, and entire lives by how well or poorly they've eaten, and they let that subject override pretty much everything else. In all areas of life, in fact, they pay much more attention to their "failures" than to their "successes."

Of note, science assures us that there is some biological basis for this common worldview: simplistically speaking, some people are blessed with happy genes and some aren't. Moreover, some people have had an upbringing in which life goes pretty smoothly, and because their parents modeled effective problem solving, they learned to manage whatever challenges come their way. Others are born with a tendency to see storm clouds on every horizon. And if they are born to parents who are downbeat or depressed, critical, anxious, or poor problem solvers, they don't get off to a very positive start in life.

We don't choose our genes; we have no choice in who our parents are, and scant power to affect our upbringing, so we come to adulthood as a composite of the heredity and socialization we received. If you were taught that problems are obstacles to pleasure, or that most of them were put there to ruin your happiness, you're certainly not going to view them as a normal part of life or as a challenge. If you were schooled to believe that your problems are worse than anyone else's, you're going to envy people who seem to have fewer of them. Moreover, if you were raised to believe that problems overshadow all the positive things in life, you're going to miss out on enjoying those positive things and insist that you're living under a permanent dark cloud.

I recall a client who really believed a nasty dark cloud chased her around. She had difficulty getting past the fact that she couldn't have children (yet she never raised the subject of possibly adopting them) and, as proof of the cloud's existence, often brought up the fact that several of her siblings had died before their time. In fact, she did have a hellacious childhood, but her current life was pretty darned good: she had an excellent job, friends, and a loving husband. By letting what she lacked dominate her thinking, she missed out on appreciating the good fortune she had.

▰▰ Get Smart!

How do you view problems — as a natural part of life or as major impediments to your pleasure and peace of mind? Is this a view your parents held? What were you taught by them about problems and problem solving? What view would you like to have about problems, and what will you do to alter your attitude?

A key skill in problem solving is holding a positive, empowering view of what happens to you in life. In fact, the word *problem* is fraught with a gloomy denotation. According to the 2014 *Oxford Dictionary* online, it means "a matter or situation regarded as unwelcome or harmful and needing to be dealt with and overcome." Ouch, huh? Embedded in this meaning is the idea that an event has appeared unbidden in order to harm us, and that we'd better fix it ASAP before it does us in. Well, that's a cheery way of looking at circumstances that are part and parcel of life.

People who appear to deal well with problems tend to see them not as impossible situations out to get them but as challenges that can be surmounted. Debris on the garden path isn't a reason to turn around and head home, but rather an occasion to figure out how to clear the path or enjoy the walk anyway. As I said, some people come by this attitude genetically or as a result of their upbringing, and it makes life hugely easier to manage. If, however, you are not one of these people, you can still, at whatever age you are now, learn to be more like them.

How? One way is through an approach called positive psychology. Even the name points you in an uplifting direction. According to Dr. Martin Seligman, director of the Positive Psychology Center, this scientific approach "has three central concerns: positive emotions, positive individual traits, and positive institutions." Here are its key points (which I've reproduced as bullet points to make them easier to absorb):

- Understanding positive emotions entails the study of contentment with the past, happiness in the present, and hope for the future.
- Understanding positive individual traits consists of the study of strengths and virtues, such as the capacity for love and work, courage, compassion, resilience, creativity, curiosity, integrity, self-knowledge, moderation, self-control, and wisdom.
- Understanding positive institutions entails the study of meaning and purpose as well as the strengths that foster better communities, such as justice, responsibility, civility, parenting, nurturance, work ethic, leadership, teamwork, purpose, and tolerance.

The goal of positive psychology is not to make you giddy or euphoric all the time or to blind you to what may harm you. It's one thing to wear rose-tinted glasses and quite another to wear no glasses at all if you need them! Rather, positive psychology maintains that we can be taught to view the world in a more optimistic manner, just as many of us were taught to view it in a pessimistic one. Suffice it to say that what you focus on in life will dictate both your worldview and how successful you are in negotiating the vicissitudes of life.

As I've maintained in this book, there is a host of skills for you to learn that can help resolve your eating problems and improve your life. Toward that end, I heartily encourage you, if you tend to be negative, critical, depressed, or a worrier, to learn more about positive psychology by examining the Positive Psychology Center's website and the many books written about the subject. Remember, one of the first steps in transformation is to change your negative thinking, because it generates pessimistic feelings. Even if you can't do a complete makeover on yourself and become a person who's always chipper and looks on the bright side, I guarantee you'll learn techniques and strategies to alter your mind-set about problems and, therefore, about problem solving.

▓ Get Smart!

Are you a pessimist or an optimist or somewhere in between? What prevents you from thinking positively and viewing problems as learning experiences or temporary impediments to success? Take a minute to consider your eating problems, and *right now* say something positive about your ability to recover.

If I Look at Problems in a Rosy Light, Will They Bloomin' Go Away?

There are two types of difficulties we all face: those that are temporary and easily resolved, and those that are more permanent and chronic — ones we must learn to live with. Being able to distinguish between the two is a crucial skill. After all, you don't want to emotionally equate getting a scratch on your brand-new car with the fact that your brother was just diagnosed with prostate cancer. But that's what some people do. They just lump all their misfortunes together and get equally upset by them all.

The good news is that some problems do go away: you have a cavity filled, and the pain in your tooth stops; your noisy neighbors move to another state; winter passes and you don't have your heart in your mouth while slipping and sliding on ice every day; and your hellion of a teenager matures into a surprisingly sweet twentysomething. The nature of these examples is that they are temporary. That doesn't mean your toothache won't return at some point, or that you won't develop pain in another tooth; that you are sure never to have troublesome neighbors again; that winter won't return; or that your congenial young adult won't occasionally exhibit the worst traits of adolescence.

It's important, when a problem is over and done with, to recognize it as such and be grateful that it's gone. But you may find yourself spending much of your time worrying that, like the shark in *Jaws*, the problem is sure to return. This is a great way of ruining good times or, worse, preventing yourself from having them. So make sure that when a problem is resolved — your computer is finally working again after crashing, your eyebrows are growing back after you burnt them off when the grill misfired, you've found a terrific new babysitter to replace the one who went off to college — that you aren't continuing to replay the things that haven't gone swimmingly. Mind that you aren't so afraid old problems will recur that you can't relax and enjoy life. If that happens, you might as well still have your original difficulties.

I see this kind of ongoing fear frequently when clients are attempting to improve their eating habits, lose weight, or generally take better care of themselves. Rather than glory in their bits of progress and feel deep pride in doing what's best for themselves even occasionally, they won't allow themselves positive feelings because they're afraid they'll lose their gains. If this isn't pretzel logic, I don't know what is. What's the point of not enjoying the present because the future might hold pain? Sure, you think you're preparing yourself for disappointment over a return engagement of misery, but what you're actually doing is trashing the here and now. Better to enjoy the pleasure sandwiched in between periods of difficulty. It makes these upbeat moments all the sweeter and gives you something to look forward to when a cloud happens to stall above your head.

Moreover, some dysregulated eaters won't permit themselves pride in taking small problem-solving steps and instead insist on waiting until all their behaviors related to food are perfect before they let themselves feel good. The truth is, they will never be perfect, because that is not what "normal" eating is all about. If you are making any kind of progress, focus on that and not on your failures.

If the good news is that some problems are temporary, the bad news is that some aren't. There are chronic health problems like irritable bowel syndrome, gum disease, migraines, arthritis, sciatica, cancers, and other recurrent conditions. Some people have thinning hair or plantar fasciitis. Others have seasonal allergies, hearing loss, or fibromyalgia. The truth is that everyone has something. True, some people have more, or worse, somethings than others, but life isn't a competition to see who can make it through with the fewest difficulties. We each have what we have.

When problems are ongoing or recurrent, it makes sense to acknowledge that fact rather than think every bout is the last. Maybe you'll be right and it will be, but don't be surprised if it isn't. And I'm not just talking about health problems. Cars and houses get old, friendships fray, and weather takes its toll. We get old and so do the items we own. And often what we call a problem is just nature doing its thing. That is *life*! This sentiment reminds me of what a therapist friend said to me once — and trust me, this woman has had a lot of ups and downs in her life. "Why," she wondered, "can't I ever get it across to my clients that things going wrong for them don't need to be a drama? It's simply the nature of existence." The more you can accept even the most devastating problems as part of what happens to human beings living on earth, the easier it will be for you to handle them.

There are two other kinds of problem categories: those that befall us through no fault of our own, and those we bring on, in whole or in part, by ourselves. And there's a mighty long continuum between the two. Dysregulated eaters tend to heap blame on themselves for their eating and weight challenges, instead of acknowledging that, although they have free will, they also are subject to the laws of heredity and to being socialized in certain ways that can't help but affect their mental and physical health. How can you accept the fact that both sets of grandparents, your parents, and all your siblings have food problems, just as you do, and that it may be more difficult for you than for other people (yet not impossible) to eat "normally"? How will you learn to live with the knowledge that sexual, emotional, or physical abuse and other kinds of trauma that you've suffered put you at risk for eating and weight struggles and how will you improve your relationship with food and your body?

One thing you can do this minute is stop blaming yourself for your eating problems. There's no point in faulting your heritage either, though it does help enormously to recognize genetic and traumatic factors. Once you accept that there is no such thing as an even playing field in life, you can acknowledge what has made you as you are and start taking responsibility for changing it. You may have to work harder than other people, it's true. But they likely will be working harder to solve some difficulty that doesn't even show up on your radar screen as a problem — and that's the way the ball bounces. Remember, even if you brought on a problem yourself, you are as entitled to fix it as you would be if it simply befell you. Who cares how it came about? It doesn't matter. The goal is to get rid of the problem, not to punish yourself by failing to do all you can to resolve it. All you need is an improved skill set. To paraphrase Albert Einstein, to solve our problems we need thinking skills better than the ones we were using when we created the problems to begin with.

 Get Smart!

Do you lump problems together as all awful, or are you able to view them according to their true threat level? Do you tend to have the same overreactions to all problems major and minor, whether they are temporary or chronic? Make a statement about how you will view problems in a more realistic light from now on. Do you feel differently about the problems you've created than about the ones that could happen to just anyone?

What Skills Do I Need for Problem Solving?

Well, first you want to have the right attitude — that is, that you will remain hopeful and try your darndest to improve a situation. No telling yourself before you begin that your efforts aren't going to work. As the saying goes, if you think you can't, you can't! So believe you can, and you will!

Even though some people seem like natural-born, terrific problem solvers, there's usually a method to their madness and many years of practice involved. Assume that you will get better at problem solving as you apply yourself, and know that you will have no shortage of difficulties to practice on.

Be Willing to Experiment

One of the first traits to develop is a willingness to experiment. Unless you're performing triple bypass surgery or are an assassin who has only one bullet to fell your elusive target, you probably have some latitude in the way you go about resolving a problem. So, the best thing you can do initially is to keep your mind open to solutions. Don't grab onto the first fix you think of, or one that is pushed on you by some well-meaning friend or know-it-all authority figure. Unless your house is on fire or your child needs to be rushed to the hospital, you're better off taking time to come up with your own plan.

Always consider various options before choosing the best of them. Noodle over solutions alone and brainstorm with people. Don't say no to any solution initially. Don't rule out what Dad says because you want to come up with a fix yourself. Conversely, don't acquiesce to what Dad says because you want to show him how much you respect his strategic abilities and garner his approval.

Don't Rush In; Step Back and Take Your Time

If you can pull back and use a wide-angle lens to view a problem, you'll see it in context. Stand too close and you may see only a small part of it. For example, if a molar hurts and gets attended to, and then the tooth next to it starts to throb, the problem might be that your bite is misaligned. If your daughter has had difficulty in every math class she's ever taken, don't simply assume she's not trying hard enough or that she has ineffective teachers. She may have significant learning disabilities.

So often we get an idea of how to solve a problem and rush out to do it. I've certainly been guilty of this approach myself. My husband, on the other hand, takes his sweet time and thinks about a problem from all angles, mentally thumbing through a host of solutions before moving forward. His tendency to be methodical and cautious has been known to drive me a mite crazy, but I'm also impressed with and immensely grateful for his effective problem-solving skills.

Reassess, Reassess, Reassess

It's useful when you're problem solving to take a break and see how things are going. A few months ago, I was trying to fix a belt buckle and kept whacking it so hard with the hammer that it broke apart. If I'd stopped after gently tapping it a few times, I would have seen that the metal was caving and about to snap. The lesson here: you don't want to approach life by whacking at your problems with a hammer!

Nowhere is it more necessary to keep evaluating how things are going than when you're trying to resolve medical problems. We tend to either go full tilt with what doctors and other medical personnel instruct us to do or insist on making ourselves better without asking for help. Instead, gather as much information as possible and make informed decisions based not on hopes and wishes but on reality and evidence. Some problems will resolve themselves and some won't. Either way, you will have done the best you could with the information you had — and that's the best that any of us can do.

Know When You're Done

Here's that pesky issue again: knowing when enough is enough. Sometimes you want to do a perfect or near perfect job when you're resolving a problem. I sure hope that my dentist feels that way when he's making me a new crown, and that my mechanic goes the whole nine yards when he's installing a new carburetor in my car. However, it doesn't always matter that a problem is solved to perfection. For instance, if you decide to throw a last-minute party, but you have barely any food in the pantry, maybe it's no big deal if, instead of preparing everything yourself, you potluck it and guests simply bring whatever they want. Similarly, if your living-room rug is permanently stained in certain areas, must you recarpet the entire room or can you get by with a few well-placed throw rugs?

Recognize Your Path to Success

One of the most important skills that expert problem solvers have is the ability to recognize what they did to solve a previous problem, so that if need be they can replicate those steps in the future. Moreover, successful problem solvers are able to generalize the steps they took that led to success. When I sat down to write my first book, *The Rules of "Normal" Eating*, the endeavor seemed daunting. I had a vague outline to work from, and the rest of the material was still in my head. My agent suggested that I develop a more detailed outline, so that is what I did. The new outline solved the problem of what I was going to write, and now I create a fairly detailed outline whenever I'm planning a book.

 Get Smart!

Which problem-solving approaches have helped you resolve difficulties? Which ones could you improve? Think about the times you've done a great job fixing problems, and identify what you did that led to success. Repeat as needed.

Unfortunately, there are several common personality traits that may get in the way of being a super-duper problem solver:

Denial

"What grinding sound in my car's wheelbase?" "No way that tree's going to fall on the house." "I still have plenty of time to get my taxes done." "It's probably not cancer, so the heck with going to the doctor." "I'm going to tell the boss what I think of her, and I don't care if she fires me." "I can quit drinking myself." "But my Uncle Sal smoked two packs a day and lived to be 103."

Well, you can tell where all these statements are heading, and it's nowhere you'd want to go. When we deny a truth that is obvious to the rest of the world, it's because we're afraid. We're not purposely trying to exacerbate our difficulties and do ourselves in. In a twisted sort of way, we're trying to take care of ourselves by avoiding heightened emotional discomfort. Denial makes a convoluted kind of sense, but it's far from life enhancing. If primitive humans had engaged in denial often enough, we wouldn't be here today.

To complicate matters, there are actually times when denial is useful.

A certain amount of denial is necessary so we can live without being constantly depressed. Who wants to think a lot about the possibility of getting Alzheimer's or a terminal illness like ALS? What would happen if you regularly thought about the fact that one day the world will be here and you won't? If every day you gazed in the mirror and said that someday you'll look so old you'd barely recognize yourself, you'd probably stop peering into the looking glass altogether.

Just remember that there's a difference between denying that fixable problems exist and being able to go with the flow when problems are irreparable.

Victim Mentality

I've already described in this book the dangers of holding on to a victim mentality, so I'll make only brief mention of it here. I'll go out on a limb and promise that you will never be a skilled problem solver if you insist on seeing yourself as a perpetual victim. Telling yourself what you can't do and why you can't do it, for whatever reason, is nothing less than marinating your mind in hopelessness and despair. It creates anxiety and negativity, which are the antitheses of the creativity you need to resolve problems. The time to see whether success is in the cards is *after* you've tried to solve the problem, not *before*. I understand that the reason you downplay the possibility of resolving your difficulties is that you don't want to be disappointed if you fail, but that's no excuse for programming yourself for failure. You allow yourself to think either like a victim or like an empowered problem solver, but you can't do both. You choose.

Chronic Fantasizing

Many dysregulated eaters fantasize a lot — and I mean a whole lot. Some spend almost as much time in their fantasies as they do in reality. Daydreaming a bit here and there — about how great life's going to be when you graduate from college, about the award ceremony for your agency, or about your upcoming Bahamian vacation with the family — is a pleasant way to pass time and often shifts your energy from negative to positive. Moreover, noodling about problems can be a creative way of dreaming up solutions. I do it often, especially when I'm trying to come up with a book title. Daydreaming in targeted, useful ways can often help solve problems.

On the other hand, chronic daydreaming, on autopilot, which I'd define as daydreaming daily or many times a week for prolonged periods of time, is nothing but an escape from reality. Studies tell us that fantasizing about what we want to happen triggers the release of dopamine in our brains. No wonder losing yourself in happy thoughts can become a habit. How much more pleasant that is than acknowledging being mired in problems. But when you're fantasizing, you're moving away from finding solutions, not toward them. So, do keep the daydreams in check. Break the habit, and put the time you'd use for it into solving your problems by becoming a critical thinker.

I Thought We Weren't Supposed to Think Critically, but Now You're Saying We Need to Learn Critical Thinking: What's Up with That?

Most people go through a lifetime without hearing or speaking the term *critical thinking*. Or, if they do use it, they're describing being critical of themselves or others. The term means nothing of the sort, but is instead a way of approaching decision making and problem solving that uses your brain to its best advantage. Experts studying critical-thinking skills use different criteria to describe this process. Attributes of critical thinkers include open- and fair-mindedness, rationality, curiosity, a desire to be well informed, flexibility, and respect for differing points of view. Robert H. Ennis offers some useful additions to this list: a person with critical-thinking skills is "capable of taking a position or changing a position as evidence dictates, [can] take the entire situation into account, [can] deal with the components of a complex problem in an orderly manner, and [can] use credible sources."

I'll add the characteristic of skepticism to the criteria listed so far. It's not to your advantage to believe everything you see or hear — such as your best friend touting her success with some weight-loss pill, a diet book on the *New York Times* bestseller list for two months that makes you want to believe the authors know what they're talking about, or an infomercial citing study after study about the wonders of some new exercise machine.

Am I getting through to you? Where is your healthy skepticism? Out the window is where. Consider what kind of critical-thinking skills your best friend has if she would use weight-loss pills; consider whether, just because a book is popular, that means it speaks the truth; and consider whether the makers of an infomercial would really go out of their way to present studies that don't support their product's success.

If you're still not getting a clear-as-day mental picture of the consummate critical thinker, it may be easier to develop an image from some of the things he or she is not: impulsive, illogical, reactive, rigid, unquestioning, afraid of being wrong, dogmatic, closed-minded, narrow-minded, irrational, a believer in pie in the sky, a Pollyanna, overly trusting, or myopic.

Hopefully, you know people who are critical thinkers, and you may even be one yourself. The truth is that people may use critical-thinking skills in one area, such as their job, but never use them anywhere else. Take a minute to tick off the attributes of critical thinkers, and see if you fit the bill.

My point in talking about this subject is that there are all sorts of ways to solve problems, including being solely intuitive, which in my experience is the wrong direction for dysregulated eaters to take, especially when it comes to their eating problems. They often say things like: "I feel fat" or "I can't stand going to the doctor." Statements like these are the antithesis of critical thinking and are among the barriers keeping troubled eaters from making progress.

If you intend to resolve your eating problems once and for all, you must develop critical-thinking skills. You can't keep wishing and hoping and thinking and praying that you're going to be a "normal" eater. You can't expect to keep making decisions and solving life's big and little difficulties, including eating problems, without them. Face it: unless you're willing to make a huge effort to change your behavior, it's going to stay the same.

Let's look at an example to see how an emotional-eating situation could play out. Say you, as a noncritical thinker, are alone at home with plenty to do and no energy to do it. The thought of munching mindlessly or having a binge has been lurking in the back of your mind all day, and you haven't been able to shake it. Rather than be curious about options you could take other than eat if you're not hungry, you stick your head into the refrigerator to see if you can find anything interesting to eat. Then, instead of taking the entire situation into account — that is, instead of recognizing that your problem has nothing to do with food and everything to do with your mood — you pull out some leftover quiche and take a forkful. Without calculating the consequences and allowing yourself to change your mind, you figure that since you already started on the quiche you should finish it, and then you'll just skip dinner. And there you have a typical scenario of acting without first employing critical-thinking skills.

Dysregulated eaters often fall short on a number of clear-thinking attributes. Rather than being curious about their behavior, they're automatically judgmental. If you've eaten an entire apple pie in a sitting (something I used to do decades ago), the mental place to go to when you're wiping the crumbs off your mouth isn't to judgment but to curiosity. Not "Shame on me for doing that" but "Why the hell did I do that?" If you can develop curiosity, that's an excellent start to critical thinking.

As noted earlier, people with food problems are often short on skepticism. They wish so desperately to lose weight — sadly, more than they want to become healthy — that they will try anything and everything that promises the pounds will fly off. It truly breaks my heart to hear of people wasting their well-earned money and precious time on bogus plans, programs, and products. Instead, look for documented, impartial studies on weight-loss methods, if you must focus on weight at all. Don't just ask your doctor, but do a lengthy and substantive search on the internet to dig up any dirt — such as lawsuits against a program or product — on whatever you intend to do. If a procedure has a low success rate, don't fall into denial and tell yourself that you're going to be one of the rare lucky ones, just because you want to be. Think of skepticism as one of the sharpest tools in your toolbox for recovery.

Please understand that I'm encouraging you to develop critical-thinking skills not only in the food arena but also in every aspect of life. Many troubled eaters agree to take on tasks without first thinking through what work is involved, then feel overwhelmed, get stressed out, and head for a Double Whopper. Remember that you can develop the skills to make informed choices so that you know exactly what you're getting into, and that you're allowed to change your mind if the evidence doesn't stack up the way you believed or were told it did.

▞ Get Smart!

Be honest, how effective are your critical-thinking skills? Which traits do you possess? Which traits do you lack? Which traits will be the most difficult to acquire? Which will most improve your relationship with food and enhance your life in general?

You know, it's funny about eating disorders. In order to recover from them, you have to mend so many of the broken parts of your life. They are a gift in that sense. Before reading this chapter, you might not have known that your problem-solving skills could use a bit of polishing up. And you might never have even considered how critical-thinking skills could improve every aspect of living.

Using intuition to help you maneuver through life is a legitimate approach. But remember that you want facts and clearheaded thinking to back up most decisions. One approach is not better than the other. The idea is to be skilled at both and know which application is necessary for which situation, and how to use one to complement the other.

Skill Boosters

1. Make a list of your irrational beliefs about "problems," and reframe them as rational beliefs. If you need help, use the beliefs section of my *Rules of "Normal" Eating*.
2. Start a pride or gratitude journal and write in it every night. Include behaviors you are proud of (no matter how inconsequential you think they are) and ones that make you glad you're you.
3. Within the next twenty-four hours, be more upbeat in two situations in which you'd normally be critical or hopeless.
4. When someone asks how you are from now on, say something positive about your life before saying something negative

(especially if the person asking is your therapist — surprise them!).

5. Listen to how you portray your life to other people. Do you describe yourself in a way that says you're a strong, kick-ass person, or in a way that says you're inadequate or a victim?

6. How did each of your parents view and manage problems? How does this influence your mind-set about your challenges today?

7. Sort through your problems and make a list of minor irritations, as opposed to major difficulties.

8. Sort through your problems and make a list of difficulties that are temporary, as opposed to chronic ones.

9. Describe the kind of attitude you'd like to have about minor, temporary problems, and what kind you wish to have about major, chronic ones.

10. Name three ways you can change in order to be more upbeat about all your problems.

11. Identify the skills you need for effective problem solving, which ones you have, and which ones you will work to acquire.

12. Name three things you enjoy (yes, enjoy) about problem solving.

13. Think of something "bad" that happened to you this week, and write a few sentences about it as if you were a victim. Then write a few sentences about the same event, taking responsibility for and empowering yourself. Do this every day with one incident.

14. Hear and watch the news with skepticism. Look for discrepancies, contradictions, and outright falsehoods. Do the same with stories people tell you that sound fishy but which they insist are true.

15. Ask people why they believe what they do, and what evidence they have to support their opinions. Always ask (nicely, of course), "How do you know that?"

16. Practice one aspect of critical thinking every day — being

curious, skeptical, seeing the whole picture, entertaining the opinion of someone with a viewpoint different from yours, changing your mind because you think someone has a better way of managing a difficult situation than you do, or insisting upon seeing or hearing evidence.

In chapter 8, you'll learn whether goal setting will benefit your unique personality and how to get the most out of goals.

CHAPTER 8

Setting and Reaching Goals

What If I Can't Get There from Here?

Dysregulated eaters are masterful at setting goals. And they're often great at reaching them as well. I've met scores of clients over the decades who've lost a hundred pounds or more several times. Maybe you've done that too. Some have lost and regained the same bleepin' twenty, thirty, or seventy-five pounds more times than they can count. People who don't have eating problems and can maintain their weight, or who lose a couple of pounds fairly easily, have no idea how difficult it is to reduce their body size in a major way and hold on to the weight loss. Most of them are clueless about the heartache and disappointment that ensue after regaining lost weight that took forever to lose.

The fact that you're reading this book suggests you have been on a diet at some point in your life. Or perhaps you have dieted all of your life and just can't seem to get anywhere. You may be close to giving up on trying to change your eating habits or shed pounds, because the time and effort just don't seem worth it, or because you now understand that diets don't work in the long term for the majority of people.

Is that because most people don't know how to set and reach their goals? Of course not. Eating healthfully and weight loss are not merely a matter of wanting something and going after it. Rather, the whole subject of our relationship with food and the number on the scale is enormously complex and depends far more on biology than on the concepts of internal control and self-discipline. According to Gina Kolata, author of *Rethinking Thin: The New Science of Weight Loss — and the Myths and Realities of Dieting*, researchers concluded from a study of identical twins, published in 1990 in the *New England Journal of Medicine*, that "70% of the variation in people's weights may be accounted for by inheritance, which means that a tendency toward a certain weight is more strongly inherited than nearly any other tendency." More recent studies, Kolata says, put weight and body-mass-index heritability closer to 65 percent. That means that about 30 percent of weight is determined by socialization, lifestyle, environment, and other nonbiological factors, one of which is life skills.

Aren't Goals Really Simple, Like, Duh, I Want to Eat Healthfully and Lose Weight?

To answer that question, let's move away from eating and weight concerns and look at goals in general for a minute. What is their purpose, and why are we so terribly attached to having and meeting them? To summarize the definitions of goals from several different dictionaries, let's say a goal is an aim, an end toward which you put effort, something you're trying to achieve. So far, so good. That's easy to understand.

But the plot thickens, because some goals are explicit — we're aware of having them — and some are implicit: we're unaware of having them. It makes sense that, in order to reach goals, we'd make them explicit, because if you don't know that you wish to do something — or how important it is to you — how are you going to motivate yourself to do it? Here's what I mean. Say you tell yourself you're going to the local bar Friday night to catch up with your friends for your weekly meet-up, but deep down your goal is to spend time with that cute redheaded guy who hangs out there, who said he'd call and never did. Well, if you don't acknowledge your desire to pursue Mr. Red Hair, you're less likely to sidle up to him at the bar and start a conversation.

Why? Because implicit goals often remain unpursued and, therefore, unattained. Maybe you don't want to admit to yourself how interested you are in Mr. Red Hair, because, after all, if he were into you, he would have called by now, wouldn't he? You're disappointed but want to pretend you're not, so you tell yourself that maybe he lost your number, has been out of town, or was kidnapped by aliens.

See what I mean? You're wishy-washy about bumping into Mr. Red Hair, can't acknowledge your desire to bump into him, and therefore likely won't make much of an effort to seek him out. But think of what you might accomplish if your goal is explicit. You might ask your friends to keep an eye out for him and let you know if he arrives, so that as naturally and normally as can be, you can mosey over and start up a conversation with him. Similarly, you might amble over to his friends and inquire about him (which would likely get back to him even if he doesn't show that night). Can you see how having an explicit goal would exponentially improve your chances of meeting Mr. Red Hair?

Returning to the subject of eating and weight, you may also have eating and weight goals that are not all that explicit. Remember that humans are very complex, and though we'd like to believe the opposite, things are not always as they seem, even within ourselves. For instance, you may tell everyone you want to lose weight *to be healthier,* which is your explicit goal, while your implicit goal is to shed twenty pounds *to be more attractive* now that you've started up a casual flirtation with a colleague. Rather than shy away from implicit goals, it's important to identify them and be honest with ourselves so we can determine whether they are realistic and compatible with our values.

▰▰ Get Smart!

Are most of your goals explicit and conscious, or are they implicit and more or less hidden from you? Take your implicit eating goals and make them explicit. Be honest!

So, along with having conscious goals, we also have unconscious ones that often trump our best intentions. Said another way, we have motivations to avoid reaching our goals as surely as we have motivations to reach them, and we must ferret out those hidden barriers in order to be successful. Clinically speaking, hidden goals are called *latent* and recognized goals are called *manifest*. As the words imply, we're usually highly conscious of a manifest goal — say, to join a gym and become fit — and not so aware of a latent goal, such as a desire to avoid adding one more activity to our already brimming schedules and stressful lives.

Here are examples of manifest (overt) and latent (covert) motivations in the eating and fitness arenas. The first part of each statement is manifest, and the second part is latent.

- You say you want to eat "normally," but, like many dysregulated eaters, you also want to continue using food to comfort yourself.

- You insist you want to go to the gym, but are ashamed of how your body looks and how little exercise you're able to do, since you're out of shape.

- You want to lose weight to be healthier, but you're anxious about slimming down because every time you've lost weight before you've been hit on sexually to the point where you almost cheated on your partner.

- When you lose weight, your friends think you look great, but you hate how your parents complain that you're too thin and, consequently, constantly try to fatten you up.

- You want to eat more nutritiously, but that means spending time you don't think you have in order to shop for, prepare, and cook foods other than those your family wants to eat.

Can you see how confounding this might be — being aware only of one set of motivations when you actually have two? Of course you have a hard time moving in one direction when you have feelings pulling you in another. No wonder you have difficulty attaining your goals or maintaining them — what you call reaching them, then backsliding. We'll talk more about this subject, along with the subjects of relapsing and self-sabotage, later on in this chapter. If you're eager to gain a greater understanding of conscious and unconscious motivations and goals, my book *Starting Monday: Seven Keys to a Permanent, Positive Relationship with Food* is all about how to identify and resolve these internal conflicts.

Get Smart!

In your own words, describe the difference between manifest and latent motivations. Give examples of goals you've failed to reach or have reached but not sustained because you've been hindered by your latent, often conflicting, motivations.

How Come Our Culture Makes Goal Setting and Achievement Seem Like a Cinch, with Oodles of Books and Seminars on the Subject?

Well, if it were such a snap, why would we need all those books and seminars? Why would you be reading this book? In theory, setting and maintaining goals is easy-peasy — just follow these steps and you'll be successful — but in practice, it can be anything but easy. I'm not saying it isn't worthwhile to set down your aims, read books on goal setting, or even have a coach spur you along. These are all valuable activities for certain people. All I'm saying is not to expect the process to be all it's cracked up to be. In my personal and professional experience, there's a whole lot more to attaining and maintaining goals than what meets the eye, especially the subtleties, described earlier, involving explicit and implicit goals. There's also what I call goal interruptus owing to latent motivations.

When I searched for "goal setting" books on Amazon.com, I came up with 68,680 results. Whew! Lots of people are certainly reaching their goal if it's to publish a book on goals! That said, let's look at some advice by goal gurus on getting where you want to go and staying there. Michael Hyatt, motivational speaker and bestselling author of *Platform: Get Noticed in a Noisy World*, a book on successful leadership in business, encourages people to do the following:

- Keep goals few in number.
- Make them "SMART," an acronym for five objectives: specific, measurable, actionable, realistic, and time-bound.
- Write them down.
- Review them frequently.
- Share them selectively.

Sounds pretty easy, doesn't it? Then we have Bradley Foster, life and executive coach, who says you need to do the following:

- Believe and have faith in the process.
- Visualize what you want.
- Get it down in writing.
- Have purpose.
- Commit to the process.
- Stay focused.
- Have a plan of action.
- Do something right now that will get you moving toward fulfilling your goals.
- Be accountable.
- Review your goals and actions taken daily.

▰▰ Get Smart!

What has been your experience with setting and reaching eating or weight goals? Is your problem one of attaining or of maintaining goals — or both? What impact have workshops or books had on your success rate?

I don't know about you, but I can't quibble with either Mr. Foster or Mr. Hyatt. I think they're both right on the money, and that what they say seems mostly like common sense, but it is also likely based on research about goals and success. The thing is, my assessment from thirty years of clinical experience flies in the face of their advice — either these techniques don't work with dysregulated eaters, or this population doesn't seek out these strategies and use them effectively. Frankly, I don't know many people, other than athletes and business executives or colleagues who are life coaches, who work with goals so specifically and comprehensively. But, I have tried assiduously to get clients to set and follow through with goals, and the process, at least as it relates to eating and self-care, simply has not worked.

For example, in my coaching and psychotherapy sessions, and in workshops, I generally ask if clients or participants want homework between sessions and I give them assignments. Often people in these settings seem eager for homework — and occasionally they even complete it. These people are often successful in life and accomplished in their fields, and they zip through a to-do list with little apparent effort. So I know they're capable of setting goals and following through. But when it comes to eating and self-care, honestly, not so much…

That is why I suggest caution when throwing yourself into goal setting in the eating, fitness, and self-care arenas, if it hasn't worked for you in the past. That doesn't mean you can't reach your goals; it just means you may want to go about achieving them in a less direct way. If you're going to rely on setting and meeting goals as your primary method of forging ahead, you had better make darn sure you aren't ambivalent about succeeding. If you insist on setting goals, you'll want to be certain you've deeply and thoroughly explored any mixed feelings you might have about being thinner or giving up food dependence.

The truth is that people who succeed with goals are generally unambivalent about reaching them. If you're going the goal route, you'd better make sure that you believe you are 100 percent worthy of success. You'd better shout out an unequivocal, resounding "Yes!" when asked if you deserve to be happy and healthy. Most dysregulated eaters answer that question with a little hemming and hawing followed by hesitant responses.

If you're going to do any goal setting — and I'm not against it — I highly recommend that you make sure you break those suckers down into manageable pieces. The biggest problem I've run into with dysregulated eaters, most of whom happen to be perfectionists, is that they're wildly out of sync with reality when it comes to setting doable goals. For example, here's what I hear: "I'll go to the gym every day after work, shop only at the farmers' market, eat organic, get the family into weekend hikes and bike rides, fit into my size-ten jeans by New Year's Eve, look awesome in my bikini for that cruise, and eat no foods that are white."

Dysregulated eaters seem to fall at either end of the spectrum: their expectations are too high and they're living on Fantasy Island, or they don't want to disappoint themselves and so they shrug off goal setting. But fear not, you can reach your goals if you're willing to go a more nontraditional route, one that is better suited to your personality and clinical issues.

All the Experts Tell Me I Must Make a Commitment to Eat Better and Exercise, So Why Can't I Just Do That and Be Done with It?

Surprisingly, one of the paths I recommend that you not take is the one where you make a commitment to be fit or eat "normally" or more healthfully. I know, I know, every book ever written about behavioral change states first and foremost that you *must* have a commitment to success. Every TV health pundit insists that you commit your heart and whatever other organs you'd care to involve in living healthfully. Well, I suggest that you look to your own experience to see if committing to a goal has worked for you. If it has, then, by all means, go the commitment route because you might succeed with it again.

However, my hunch is that your answer to my question about your success will be rather circular: that things went well while you were committed, but then they stopped going well and you were no longer committed — or you stopped being committed, so things stopped going well. So which came first, quitting the behavior or giving up the commitment? Kinda chicken-and-egg, don'tcha think?

My problem with encouraging dysregulated eaters to make commitments to become healthier comes from my decades of experience, my personal recovery from food problems, and from an understanding of why we make commitments. Evidence points to the fact that we push ourselves to commit to goals for eating, exercise, education, financial security, and so on in order *to overcome our valid doubts that we'll succeed*. Commitment portends (or, rather, pretends) certainty of our success. It feels like holding a guarantee in your hand.

But think about the concept of pledging a rigid allegiance to fitness and healthy eating. Why would we need to do that? Why wouldn't we think enough of ourselves to do what's good for us because it makes no sense to live any other way? That's the crux of the problem. My take is that we feel a need to make commitments precisely because we don't value ourselves enough to automatically do what's in our best interest.

Moreover, consider how dysregulated eaters often equate healthy and "normal" eating with restriction and deprivation. So when they commit to a "better" kind of eating, it feels like saying no to themselves a million times over. Frankly, most dysregulated eaters equate the word *commitment* with doing something arduous and distinctly unpleasant — something they don't really want to do. This association is so strong that a commitment to almost anything healthy becomes both prohibitive and sure to self-destruct sooner or later. Think about it: if eating better or becoming fitter weren't perceived as odious, we'd just do it and wouldn't have to make a commitment to it. Read on and you'll see why making promises hasn't worked for you, even when you thought you were making them for all the right reasons.

There are several reasons why making commitments doesn't work. First, *we don't make commitments to goals that make sense and that we know are easily achievable*. There's no need to. If it's easy and sensible, no big deal, we just go ahead and do it. Instead, *we make commitments to things we don't know are possible but hope or wish were*. For example, custom aside, uncertainty is the reason we may feel a need to "commit" to marriage: Because we can't see into the future and *know* we'll live happily ever after, we make a pledge in order to convince ourselves that this will be sure to happen. The same goes for diets. We have no assurance that we'll stay on them long enough for them to slim us down, so we believe with all our might (against scientific evidence and our own hard-core experience and better judgment) that our dreams of dieting down to a lower weight will come true.

Second, *the more we sacrifice for a commitment and the harder it is to keep it, the more committed we become*. Counterintuitive, huh? In terms of dieting, the more rigid a diet is — fasting, grapefruit, only carbs, no carbs, ice cream only, and so on — the stronger we cling to the belief that it's a winner. The more we must deny ourselves, the harder we try to do so, and the firmer becomes our resolve to keep on truckin'. It's true: in its own warped way, hardship strengthens commitment. Apparently we believe that whatever comes naturally and easily and makes perfect sense is not worth pursuing; but tell us the odds of success are slim to none, and you can sign us up.

Third, *the more we invest in commitments* (in the case of diets, this means time, money, energy, and constantly focusing on them), *the more difficult it is to be honest and fess up that whatever we're doing isn't working*. Instead, because we hate to think we've failed, and that we were wrong all along, and because we rue the lost time, energy, and money we've expended, we redouble our efforts and blindly soldier on.

Many dysregulated eaters say they hate dieting, but it's so ingrained in them that they still cling to remnants of a diet mentality, albeit one buried deeply below consciousness. I've worked with people for months or years on "normal" eating, only to have them tell me out of the blue that they've returned to Weight Watchers or resumed counting calories. I understand how difficult it is to give up diet thoughts, and it's precisely for this reason that I recommend not making a commitment to any kind of eating. *The act of committing*, with all its previous, negative associations, cited earlier, is going to come back and bite you.

Commitment does not forecast success. After all, look at the millions of people (maybe you) who year after year take a pledge on New Year's Day to lose weight — and fail. What does this tell you about commitments and success? Knowing dysregulated eaters as I do, I suspect that you probably think *you're* the failure. Not true! The truth is that we succeed at healthful living for other reasons; certainly not because we've made a commitment to do so. And sometimes making the commitment itself is what steers us off course.

▛▜ Get Smart!

How have you fared when you've made a commitment to eat healthfully or get fit? When commitment hasn't led to permanent success, what has gotten in the way? How do you feel about making health commitments now? What, other than commitment, might lead you to success?

Okay, So If I Don't Work toward Goals or Make a Commitment, How the Heck Am I Ever Going to Move Forward?

With baby steps, of course — as if there's any other way. There's a big difference between pushing yourself to meet a series of goals or objectives within a time frame and having a general purpose and inching toward it slowly but surely. For example, which of the following sounds more doable? Setting a goal to be a totally "normal" eater four weeks from now, or reading books on intuitive eating, joining a support group for dysregulated eaters, honestly examining why you might be a bit uneasy about slimming down or giving up food for comfort, and developing skills for living without abusing food?

In the first instance, you're focusing solely on behavior and diving in, fears and conflicting emotions be damned. In the second, you're getting your feet wet and choosing activities that will actually speed your recovery and have a huge payoff down the road. Baby steps involve *thinking* differently about eating and fitness, not simply *acting* differently.

Here are some questions to answer regarding your baby-stepping journey.

- What are valid measurements and markers of progress?
- How will I take a positive view of setbacks, mistakes, relapses, and failures?
- How will I prevent perfectionism from getting in the way of feeling good about minor achievements when I stall and plateau for a while?
- How will I progress at my own pace and ignore external pressures that make me want to move faster than is good for me?
- What life skills do I want to improve while also changing my food and fitness attitudes and habits?
- How will I make sure I get support in becoming and staying healthy?
- What functional beliefs must I have in order to take ongoing, excellent care of myself?

All these questions may seem too inconsequential to bother with, and answering them may seem like sidetracking if you are going the goal route, but I can assure you that in order to succeed in permanently caring for your body, you will need to grapple with them all and come out the other side. Let me help you answer some of these questions.

What Are Valid Measurements and Markers of Progress?

For starters, here are three concrete, simple ways to mark and measure progress. The first is by the *duration* of the dysfunctional behavior — that is, how long it goes on. Say, for example, your usual binge lasts for two hours. Or, conversely, let's say that you can starve yourself for several hours, but remain in denial that you are doing so. You're making progress in the first instance if you binge for twenty minutes, catch yourself, then stop, and in the second instance if you feed yourself nourishingly after an hour of self-imposed starvation rather than hold out for several more.

A second way to assess progress is through *intensity* — that is, how thoroughly absorbed you become in a dysfunctional behavior. Let's say, for example, that your binges are generally ferocious, and only after you've cleaned out all the food in your home do you realize you've been gorging; or that you're so totally in the grip of obsessing about weight loss that you're light-headed from not eating all day. You're making progress in the first case if, during your binge, you remain aware that what you're doing is self-destructive and you don't go totally "unconscious" and deny it. In the second case, you're inching forward if you struggle with whether or not to eat, even if you lose the debate and continue to abstain.

The third way to measure progress is by the *frequency* of undesired behavior. Maybe you now can go weeks between binges. Maybe you used to count the calories in every morsel that went into your mouth, and now you do it only after you've overeaten. The goal is to lengthen the periods of normalcy and functional behavior between bouts of dysfunction. The more you stretch out the time between incidents of dysregulated eating, the more you're retraining your brain to reregulate your appetite appropriately.

Use these markers to recognize whether you're making progress. Don't let one eating experience that you're unhappy with — or even a few — make you believe that your behavior hasn't changed at all. Look for changes in duration, intensity, and frequency to chart your movement toward recovery.

How Will I Take a Positive View of Setbacks, Mistakes, Relapses, and Failures?

One way is through the concept of "failing forward," which means using mistakes or failures in the service of moving ahead. Whereas *relapse* connotes slipping backward, failing forward is about making progress. Think of every failure to become a functional eater as preparation for success — a practice session, rehearsal, dry run, or experiment. Recognize that locked away in every error (or relapse, if you will) are all the nuggets of wisdom you need in order to not make the same error again. If you analyze why you've failed, you'll know exactly what not to do next time and what you must do to succeed in the future.

By staying with the process and doing what has proven universally effective in learning to eat "normally," you *will* reach your goals. Ironically, overfocusing on goal attainment is one of the ways you're almost certain to fail. Stop asking yourself, "How come I don't get this yet? Why am I still overeating? What's the matter with me that I'm not succeeding?" It's better to say, "This is a challenging process for everyone; I'm learning as fast as I can." Or: "I'll get there if I pay attention to what I need to learn right this minute, not push myself to recover faster." Please remind yourself that you are not in the recovery Olympics!

Another instructive way to look at progress and change — and mistakes and setbacks — is from a "fixed" versus "growth" mind-set. People with a fixed mind-set see themselves and their attributes or inadequacies as more or less permanent — they're good at some things and bad at others, outgoing or shy, lovable or unlovable, smart or stupid, period. Fixed-mind-set thinkers view their successes as the result of their positive qualities, and their failures as the result of their inherent defects. And dysregulated eaters seem to think they have a great many defects. You likely have a fixed mind-set: you're either this or that, and mostly you don't even feel good enough about yourself at your very best. Desperate to succeed, you're thrilled and relieved when you do, and you feel devastated when you don't, as if failure confirms your worst fear — that there's something permanently defective about you. Nonsense! It's all in your thinking and has nothing to do with inherent gifts or deficits.

Step outside yourself for a moment and slip into a growth mind-set. People with a growth mind-set think in terms of learning and changing to solve problems. They don't believe there's anything especially defective about them that prevents them from happiness or success. They assume that changing their attitude or behavior will resolve most problems. A fixed mind-set considers binges and overeating as by-products of character flaws, while a growth mind-set considers them as less-than-effective ways to solve problems that have nothing to do with food.

Here's another example. If you had a fixed mind-set and skipped out on going to the gym for the second time this week, you'd probably say to yourself, "What's wrong with me? I don't go because I'm lazy or unmotivated." Thinkers with a growth mind-set, on the other hand, would acknowledge the need to develop better strategies for being more active, because the ones they've been using clearly aren't working well. They would never think of attributing a lack of success to *who they are*. Rather, they'd see about changing *what they did*. Get the difference? Not to belabor the point, but a fixed-mind-set thinker would view failure as "proof that there's something wrong with me," while a growth-mind-set thinker would view it as "proof that I have yet to find better ways to succeed." If you believe you can't go from being a fixed- to a growth-mind-set thinker, then tell me: is that thought fixed or growth-oriented?

▚ Get Smart!

What has prevented you from seeing your instances of progress, however small? What ways will you change so that you can see more of your growth, rather than your lack of it? How can you develop a growth, rather than a fixed, mind-set?

How Will I Prevent Perfectionism from Getting in the Way of Feeling Good about Minor Achievements When I Stall and Plateau for a While?

Examine your beliefs about perfectionism, success, and failure, and they will give you all the information you need to abolish the desire for perfection. Perfectionism is the result of all-or-nothing thinking: if I'm not this, I must be that. But life is rarely all one way or another. Look around and decide: does life really exist only at extremes, or is there a great deal of something in between? Perfectionism, according to my colleague Joanna Poppink, author of *Healing Your Hungry Heart*, is a way to keep yourself safe and above reproach, as if by staying in the perfect zone you can prevent others from ever faulting you.

But the fact is, chasing perfection is a fool's errand. Maybe as a child you tried to be perfect to please others or to avoid mistreatment, rejection, or abandonment. Now, however, you get to evaluate yourself rather than depend on how others view you. As an adult, you're no longer at the mercy of someone else's critical standards. You can eat however you want (well or poorly) and act however you wish (again, well or poorly), and you are accountable only to yourself.

By forgoing perfectionism and making a big deal out of minor achievements, you spur yourself on. Isn't it a delicious feeling to be your own best friend and head cheerleader? And so what if you stay a while at a plateau without gaining skills or losing weight? We need to rest and consolidate changes once in a while. It's only in fantasy that change happens overnight and marches straightforward without resting. Think of a plateau as a reconsolidation spot and jumping-off place, from which you'll take your next big leap forward.

How Will I Progress at My Own Pace and Ignore External Pressures That Make Me Want to Move Faster Than Is Good for Me?

Do you ask someone else when to schedule your annual checkup, or how fast you want to be driving? Then why would you think that any individual could possibly determine your proper pace as you recover from eating problems? Who knows you best? Why, you do, of course. When you feel this kind of pressure, ask yourself why someone else wants you to speed up or slow down. If the thought comes from them, then even if your name is attached to it, how could it possibly be about anyone else but them? Remember that people — even those who profess to love you — have various reasons for wanting you to do or not do things, but that doesn't mean these reasons are in your best interest.

Other pressures may appear to be external, but they're really coming from you. Usually this pressure arises in the form of a date or event at which you want to look a certain way — thinner. You believe that people will like or value you more in a slimmer body, and that they'll be less likely to accept you the way you are. You think you'll be judged by your size. Well, the truth is that maybe you will be, and maybe you won't be; but when it comes down to it, who's the harshest critic of your appearance, hands down? I'd say it's the person whose face you see in the mirror every day. You're on yourself 24/7 about getting that new body as fast as possible. So, forget about external and internal pressures to go faster than you possibly can. Be grateful you're moving slowly. Research tells us repeatedly that gradual learning and change is the best kind. And I'll add that it's the only kind that works!

What Life Skills Do I Want to Improve While Also Changing My Food and Fitness Attitudes and Habits?

All the skills taught in this book, and whatever additional ones you want to become more proficient in, will, if practiced, speed you on your way to taking better care of your health. Maybe you want to learn to be more assertive or to take things less personally. Could that possibly hurt? Perhaps you'd like to be more outgoing, or you yearn to uncover your creative side. These skills will complement your desire to become your own person and be more fulfilled.

If I tell you now all the skills you'll need in order to live your best life, I'll be ruining all your fun. I'd rather you enjoy discovering them by yourself!

How Will I Make Sure I Get Support in Becoming and Staying Healthy?

These days there's no shortage of ways to gain support. Now that eating disorders are talked about openly in lectures and on talk shows, and binge eating has its own diagnosis in the 2013 *Diagnostic and Statistical Manual of Mental Disorders*, dysregulated eating has really taken a step out of the closet. Because of this, there's no shortage of places to get support. Of course, you can start by talking about your food problems with your friends and family, but only if you get the feeling they'll be interested and supportive. Test the waters, and don't expect everyone to understand what you're going through. Some will and some won't, and that's fine.

Think like an adult and accept that some people will want to know about your food struggles, while others will be totally uninterested or uncomfortable with the subject. Don't push. Try to educate them, and determine how educable they are. You never know if people might change their minds down the road and come around to supporting you. Alternatively, if they're not interested in what you have to say right now, so be it. Find someone who is.

Beyond seeking help from friends and family, use the skill of valuing yourself enough to check your community and online for places to share and continue growing. Be absolutely determined to get help, because you deserve it. Learning to seek help and accepting it can be major obstacles for dysregulated eaters who feel they must cure themselves alone or are too ashamed to ask for assistance. If this has been a problem for you, go out of your way to garner support and join the rest of the world in learning the joys of dependence and interdependence.

What Functional Beliefs Must I Have in Order to Take Ongoing, Excellent Care of Myself?

There are far too many such beliefs to list in the space of this book. Fortunately, I wrote *The Rules of "Normal" Eating*, which contains several chapters on rational and irrational beliefs about food, eating, weight, and body image. Moreover, the book provides instruction on and a template for changing beliefs so that you can easily learn the process for doing so.

By the way, make sure not only to develop a set of functional beliefs about eating and weight but also to pay attention to your core beliefs, which are about who you are, your place in the world, and your views of how life works. Too many people spend time reframing their food- and body-related beliefs, but leave their irrational core beliefs untouched, then wonder why they still have eating problems. The answer is that they continue to have a dysfunctional way of viewing the world and their place in it, and their food and body-image problems won't resolve until their core beliefs are healthy and rational.

A few last words about the "self" skills you'll need in order to reach the finish line. One invaluable skill is self-reflection, which means thinking often about life and everything in it, including yourself. I don't mean being self-absorbed, but wondering about your thoughts, feelings, and behaviors in a curious, nonjudgmental way. Self-reflection is the opposite of self-judgment, at which most dysregulated eaters excel. It's a neutral appraisal that you undertake in order to gather information, like listening to the news. You don't turn on CNN to like or dislike what you hear, do you? You turn it on to learn what's going on. The purpose of reflection is to get to know yourself better and then, if you wish, to apply what you learn to improving yourself.

Another essential skill is self-honesty, which is seeing not only what you've done wrong but also what you've done right. Believe it or not, this is a tall order for most troubled eaters. Most people would rather focus on their strengths, not their weaknesses. Not dysregulated eaters; they're just the opposite. So remember that being honest means it's okay that you did better than someone else, or that you were right when others were wrong, or that you were smarter, or faster, or more clever, or more successful. Excelling often makes dysregulated eaters wildly uncomfortable. While craving praise, they don't feel they deserve it or are convinced that if people really knew them, they wouldn't be praising them. They believe they're not as good as others think they are and feel like imposters. Just remember that being better (like being worse, for that matter) than someone else is almost always a temporary condition. Enjoy it for the moment, then let it go, but please don't miss out on it.

Last but not least is the essential skill of self-talk. People who are skilled in positive self-talk possess one of the greatest gifts in the world. And I don't mean giving yourself praise when you don't deserve praise, but being there for yourself every minute of every day and giving yourself whatever you need: comfort, a small dose of reality, an inner smile of encouragement, a good laugh at yourself, respect, compassion, a pat on the back for a job well done, and so on. Practice positive self-talk, especially with an eye toward compassion, and you'll be amazed that you can still be the same person but feel like a completely different one. Moreover, you will not succeed at permanently taking effective care of your health and your body if you do not become proficient at positive self-talk.

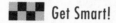 **Get Smart!**

Which of the skill areas that I've described will be easiest for you to learn? Which will be most difficult? Are there other life skills you'd like to learn in order to help resolve your eating problems? What are three positive statements that you could make about yourself right now?

Skill Boosters

1. What goals have you been successful in reaching? Was that because you did everything right to reach them, or did you reach them in spite of making mistakes along the way?
2. How successful have you been in making — or breaking — commitments?
3. What are the three markers of making progress?
4. Describe a mistake you made that turned out to be fortuitous in the long run.
5. Describe a success that you achieved by taking baby steps.
6. As if you're talking to an eight-year-old, explain why perfection is an illusion.
7. Describe pros and cons of (1) asking for support and (2) receiving support.
8. Is your mind-set fixed or growth-oriented? Explain the difference between the two.
9. Come up with a mantra to use when you or other people pressure you to move faster in your recovery than you can. (Hint: mine is "I'm doing the best I can.")
10. Make a list of irrational beliefs about being successful, needing to be perfect, getting support, needing others' approval of your eating habits or weight, and valuing yourself, then rewrite them all so they're rational (read *The Rules of "Normal" Eating* for help).
11. What are you afraid you'll see if you're honest with yourself?

How can you make it all right to see yourself honestly? (Hint: think curiosity, not judgment.)

12. At the end of every day, look back and identify something you did well and something you didn't.

13. Keep a journal that chronicles your eating progress, with a heavy emphasis on the achievements you're proud of.

14. What are the kindest, most loving and compassionate words you can say to yourself? Say them now aloud in front of a mirror. Repeat as necessary.

In chapter 9, you'll learn the purpose of work and play and how to value both.

CHAPTER 9

Balancing Work and Play

All Work and No Play Makes Jack...
Crave a Snack!

Dysregulated eaters too often spend their lives racing against the clock and can't wait until they have time to themselves. But then, more often than not, they don't know what to do with it. Busy bees, they go from dawn 'til dusk ticking off tasks on their voluminous to-do lists; and when they finally do get a chance to sit down and relax, their minds continue to torment them with what they haven't yet done and all the things they must do tomorrow. Relaxation doesn't feel right if there are chores left undone, but then, neither does doing them. Funny how the only thing that fits the bill is — guess what! — eating. After all, the thinking goes, one has to eat, doesn't one?

Is this drudge of a life the one you're living? I understand that money must be made, children demand care, and other various and sundry attentions must be paid to objects animate and inanimate. Cars require tune-ups, feet need new shoes, and living quarters require cleaning. Relatives insist on sharing your time, and lawns don't mow themselves. There is always work to do, I'll grant you that. That is, there's always work to do unless you have the financial wherewithal to pay someone to do most of it. The truth is, however, that many fortunate people who do have the money to pay others to take care of what they don't care to do still have difficulty kicking back.

So, if it's not a lack of means that prevents you from turning off your overloaded mind and resting your weary body, what is it? Could it be something within that's like a gun to your head that keeps you on the go? Could it be the guilt that pops up the minute your fanny hits the recliner, or the shame that descends on you because you feel you're being selfish by taking care of yourself? In my experience, guilt and shame are what make it difficult for dysregulated eaters to take a break and engage in what I'd call rest or play.

To play is to be engrossed in activity that has no purpose other than to bring you in-the-moment pleasure. The 2014 *Oxford Dictionary* online tells us that play is to "engage in activity for enjoyment and recreation rather than for a serious or practical purpose."

Sounds good to me! According to the National Institute for Play (who even knew there was such a thing?), play

> is a state of being that is intensely pleasurable. It energizes and enlivens us. It eases our burdens, renews a natural sense of optimism and opens us up to new possibilities. These wonderful, valuable qualities are just the beginning of what play is.
>
> Scientists — neuroscientists, developmental biologists, psychologists, scientists from every point on the scientific compass — have recently begun viewing play as a profound biological process.
>
> They are learning that play sculpts our brain; it makes us smarter and more adaptable. For many animal species it has evolved over eons with the result that the most advanced animals play the most, i.e., play is more central to their development. Humans are the biggest players of all, specially designed by nature to play throughout our long lives.

Who'd have thunk it, huh? If you hadn't read the preceding quote, would you have believed that play is an essential component of this thing we call life? Would you have known it was so valuable and vital to pleasure and happiness? If not, that's okay. By reading this chapter and following its suggestions, you'll learn to bring yourself to a higher level of enjoyment, as well as a deeper one, by developing new habits of play, passion, and pleasure.

Remember how as a child you'd go to the beach and lose yourself for hours building an elaborate sand castle with moats and turrets? Maybe you were so absorbed in your architectural endeavor that you were willing to forgo swimming or collecting shells along the seashore with your siblings. No one was paying you to build castles, but you did it anyway. And then, when you were done with your masterpiece, what did you do — after you showed it off, of course? You knocked it down and started over, building another castle. So, pray tell, was that work or play?

Many troubled eaters have difficulty with both concepts. When they're at work, they're daydreaming about having fun or kicking back, and when they're supposed to be out having a good time or enjoying relaxation, they're feverishly worrying about work. And by that, I don't mean simply that they worry about the job they're paid to do, but also that they worry about the general tasks, chores, errands, and grunt work that make up — and, sadly, take up — much of our lives. They have difficulty keeping their minds on work because they feel undervalued, taken advantage of, disinterested in what they're doing; long to be doing another activity; or resent the time spent working when they want to be playing. This makes for very unhappy and dissatisfied campers.

On the other hand, when they do finally get a chance to play or chill out, they feel guilty and can't quite let themselves go completely, because *not* enjoying themselves is a kind of penance they believe they deserve to pay for not being busy and productive. Honestly, did you have any idea that the subject of play would be so complex? Dysregulated eaters often have this kind of push-pull, confounding, tension-riddled relationship with work and play. And the reason I want to set the record straight is because I want you to develop the skill of knowing how to distinguish when it's time to work and when it's time to play, so that you can find a better balance between the two. This skill is touched on in chapters 4 and 6, so it's worth rereading them both if you suspect that being unskilled in balancing work and play is a barrier to enjoying a positive relationship with food.

▰▰ Get Smart!

What are your feelings about work and about play? How does my description of play — as necessary in order for you to thrive — change your view of it? Are you starting to understand how feeling guilty about play and relaxing drives you to eat?

If It's Natural for Children to Play, How Come I'm So Confused about the Subject?

You're not alone. Many people are unsure how much to work and how much to play. They either want to party, party, party or keep their noses to the grindstone and never look up. Any guesses on how we develop into one type of person or the other?

Although play comes naturally to children, they also enjoy learning; and without a doubt, the desire to move toward mastery is embedded in human DNA. Of course, children don't know that they're often learning while they're playing. That's the magic of play. Remember those sand castles I was talking about earlier? Consider what you learned by trial and error as you were building and rebuilding them. You learned to gauge how far back in the sand to build your castle to make sure a wave didn't roll over it and wash it away. You figured out a workable ratio of sand to water that would enable the sand to hold its shape — too little water and the sand wouldn't firm up and grains would roll or fly off, but too much and the sand would collapse into mush.

I'm sure you didn't realize at the time that you were acquiring the basics of engineering and physics as you built your dream fortress, yet you were. Moreover, even as you were finding pleasure in the mere act of fashioning your castle, you were also feeling joy in improving at what you were doing. Without your realizing it, each castle you made was likely an improvement on the last. In this way, our brains link play to learning; or to put it another way, they link fun to mastery.

But let's back up and see what would have happened if you had been messing with sand and water and having a grand old time and some well-meaning adult (a parent, relative, family friend, or even a stranger) strolled over and started instructing you on how to build a proper castle — add more water, mix in more sand, put in a drawbridge, make those turrets taller, and so on. If this person offered suggestions in a friendly, take-it-or-leave-it manner, you might have been happy that he or she had the time and interest to share ideas, and thrilled that the advice made your castle-building easier and improved the structure.

If, on the other hand, this person told you or implied that you had no idea how to build a castle, you might have felt like burying your head in the sand. If Mr. or Ms. Critical continued to drone on with unsolicited advice as if you were competing for an international architectural prize, you might have wanted to smash the whole edifice down with your fists, give up, and walk away. Worse, you might have begun to feel that play must be done in a certain way or it wasn't worth the effort. And all too likely, the joy of being in the moment and using your imagination would have washed away like the tide.

In order to understand your skill deficit in balancing work and play, you'll have to time-tunnel back to your childhood, and sort out how your parents viewed these activities, what they taught you explicitly and, perhaps more important, implicitly about them. Your responses to the following twelve statements will give you a clearer picture of your family values regarding work and play.

Exercise

1. Three words Mom might have applied to work or chores are
   _____, _____, _____.

2. Three words Mom might have applied to play or relaxing are
   _____, _____, _____.

3. Three words Dad might have applied to work or chores are
   _____, _____, _____.

4. Three words Dad might have applied to play or relaxing are
   _____, _____, _____.

5. Other significant relatives had this to say about play or being
   productive: _____

   _____.

6. One or both of my parents were overly focused on getting things done and had difficulty kicking back. ___yes ___no

7. One or both of my parents valued productivity over nonproductivity. ___yes ___no

8. Play and work were equally encouraged by my parents. ___yes ___no

9. One or both of my parents were much more interested in play than work. ___yes ___no

10. My parents enjoyed a healthy balance between work and play. ___yes ___no

11. My parents often interrupted my play or downtime with directives about getting more important things done. ___yes ___no

12. My parents taught me to enjoy a healthy balance between work and play. ___yes ___no

What did you learn from this exercise? Does it help you understand why you're not more skilled at balancing work and play? Please understand that your parents didn't set out to mess with your mind in these areas. They learned from their parents, who learned from their parents, and so on, to the beginning of your lineage. Different historical periods influenced how work and play were viewed, and class, culture, and religion had a bearing on these activities, as well. If your ancestors were landed gentry and able to afford servants, they passed down values to subsequent generations that differ from the values you inherited if you had a family tree of farmers and day laborers.

▰▰ Get Smart!

What is your understanding now of why you are unskilled at balancing work and play? Write the adage you've been living by with each of them. Write the adage you wish to live by with each of them.

Okay, So I Haven't Gotten Work and Play Exactly Right; How Do I Find a Better Balance?

I'm going to make the assumption here, based on the troubled eaters I've treated for decades, that your difficulty in discerning how to balance work and play stems from the fact that you were taught to value the former over the latter. That is, you learned by word or deed that play is a distraction or a luxury, and that it's better to work and be productive than to slack off and have a good time. This may not be true for all dysregulated eaters, but I bet it's true for many. Of course, the opposite may be true as well, that your parents goofed off a lot and didn't work very hard or teach you to do so.

Since we've been examining how your upbringing shaped your view of work and play, let's do another exercise, one that will bring your dilemma into sharper focus. Because cognitive-behavioral theory tells us that our behaviors are rooted in our beliefs, it's time to put beliefs under a microscope and examine them more closely. What you believe about work and play, even if you're unaware of these beliefs (*especially* if you're unaware of them), will dictate how you value spending your time.

First, a word about beliefs in general. Although our feelings and behaviors are based firmly on our beliefs, generally we hardly ever think seriously about them. Sure, you might pause to consider your religious beliefs when the issue of separation of church and state comes up, or ponder your convictions about child rearing when you learn you're pregnant. But for the most part, our cognitions interest us far less than our emotions and behaviors. However, in order to live a conscious life — and have a relationship with food that is positive and healthy — we *must* examine why we act and feel the way we do. I agree with Socrates who insists, "The unexamined life is not worth living." Not if you're looking to have a successful, happy, meaningful time on earth.

Now is the time to examine your irrational, dysfunctional, or otherwise unhealthy beliefs about work and play. I've corralled a bunch of beliefs on the subject in a list that follows. Some are learned from our culture through school and religion, but most are acquired from our parents and extended family.

Once more, let me assure you that I'm not blaming your parents for teaching you a set of beliefs that aren't functional. Nor am I blaming you for holding these assumptions. We all learn beliefs in childhood that don't do us proud in adulthood. The enlightened among us know this and periodically sift through our cognitions to determine if they're keepers or not. There's nothing wrong with discarding old beliefs, mind you, and selecting ones that make more sense to you nowadays. Being selective about beliefs is a sign of wisdom.

Here's one more caution: please don't judge yourself for having a belief that, said aloud, seems silly, bizarre, or otherwise unacceptable. No judgments, okay? Instead, allow yourself to be curious and completely open to whatever responses you have. Nonjudgmental self-acceptance is an essential life skill in itself and one that is sorely needed by most troubled eaters. So, here are beliefs about *work* and *play*, which are also code words for *productivity* and *relaxation*:

1. It is important, above all else, to be productive in life.
2. I can't play until I'm finished with all of my work.
3. Play is frivolous and a waste of time.
4. One of the worst things I can do is waste time.
5. If I don't stay busy, I'll get myself into trouble.
6. If I don't have anything to do, I probably left a job undone or poorly done.
7. I can play only if I squeeze it in between periods of work.
8. If I don't have goals and work toward them, I won't amount to anything.
9. I'd better keep my mind busy.
10. Adults don't have time to play; only children do.
11. There is no point in play.
12. Play only distracts me from tasks at hand.
13. To feel proud of myself, I must keep busy and be productive.
14. If I play too much, I'll never be successful.
15. If I take time off to play, people will think I'm lazy.
16. Work builds character, while play leads to shirking responsibility.
17. If there's work to be done, playing is selfish and foolish.

18. People will judge me by how much work I do and how well I do it.
19. Serious people spend time working, not playing.
20. If I haven't worked hard, I don't deserve to play.

Do any of these beliefs resonate with you? Maybe you've known all along that your ideas about work and play were a little off, but you didn't want to "waste time" thinking about them. Maybe your beliefs have made you uncomfortable and angry at your parents for instilling them in you. Perhaps you are angry at yourself for knowing that how you think is killing you little by little, but you're still living as if they're worthwhile. No matter. Set your beliefs aside and reframe them, and then you can choose which ones you want to keep. And remember, you can always change your beliefs if you get more or different information that challenges them. I hope you recall learning this in chapter 7, which lists, as a criterion for critical thinking, the ability to alter your thinking in response to new information.

Here's how I would reframe the preceding list of irrational beliefs. Feel free to "play" with them to make them truer for you.

1. It is important, above all else, to be productive in life. → Work and play are equally important.
2. I can't play until I'm finished with all of my work. → I can play whenever I want.
3. Play is frivolous and a waste of time. → Play is essential to health and well-being.
4. One of the worst things I can do is waste time. → Time is mine to do anything I want with it.
5. If I don't stay busy, I'll get myself into trouble. → I'll enjoy myself if I'm not busy.
6. If I don't have anything to do, I probably left a job undone or poorly done. → If I don't have anything to do, it's time to play.
7. I can play only if I squeeze it in between periods of work. → I can play whenever I feel like it.
8. If I don't have goals and work toward them, I won't amount to anything. → To be a fully rounded person, I need goals, work, and play.

9. I'd better keep my mind busy. → Nothing bad will happen if my mind isn't busy.

10. Adults don't have time to play; only children do. → People can enjoy play at any age.

11. There is no point in play. → The point of play is to have pleasure and fun and to unwind.

12. Play only distracts me from tasks at hand. → Play recharges me so I can return to tasks at hand.

13. To feel proud of myself, I must keep busy and be productive. → I am as proud of playing as of working and being productive.

14. If I play too much, I'll never be successful. → I can balance work and play and be successful.

15. If I take time off to play, people will think I'm lazy. → Taking time off to play is natural, healthy, and essential.

16. Work builds character, while play leads to laziness and shirking responsibility. → Play builds pleasure and sometimes new learning.

17. If there's work to be done, playing is selfish and foolish. → Taking care of myself with play is never selfish or foolish.

18. People will judge me by how much work I do and how well I do it. → I value myself for how well I balance work and play.

19. Serious people spend time working, not playing. → I can be serious sometimes and enjoy play at other times.

20. If I haven't worked hard, I don't deserve to play. → I deserve to play whether I've worked hard or not.

What did you learn from reframing your beliefs about work and play? I wouldn't be surprised if you were a tad uncomfortable in the process of reading my reframed beliefs. That's because even though you might be drawn to these new ideas, you haven't quite put your old beliefs to rest yet. That's understandable. You've had them for a long, long time, and in fact they are deeply grooved in your neural pathways. However, don't worry: as you read and act on your new beliefs repeatedly — and really think about how they belong to the person you wish to be and are becoming — they'll take root.

■■■ **Get Smart!**

How did you feel reading over the irrational, unhealthy beliefs?
How did you feel reading over the rational, healthy beliefs? What
is your next step in creating a functional belief system as a foun-
dation for work and play?

Sometimes When I'm Thinking about Food or Eating Mindlessly, I Wonder If It's Because I'm Trying to Feed My Empty Life

Dysregulated eaters are full of intriguing paradoxes. On the one hand,
their lives are overflowing and they never seem to have a moment to
spare. Then, when they do, they often feel uneasy about what to do with
it. Clients will describe eating when they feel overwhelmed and stressed
from what they perceive as too much to do, but will also cite instance after
instance when they're feeling bored and head for the fridge to do *something*. Mind-boggling indeed.

Part of the problem here has to do with self-regulation gone awry
and with getting caught up in doing too much or too little. If having too
much on your metaphoric plate triggers overeating, well, then, make sure
you do less. And if having nothing to do drives you up a wall — one that
happens to have a kitchen cabinet built into it — don't let yourself get into
that situation. But doing more or less isn't really the whole story. At the
core is your fear of an empty mind and an empty life, bereft of meaning,
attachments, and pleasure. It's the void that gets to you and that you try to
fill with food. However, you can't fill emotional emptiness with something
you chew and swallow.

There is likely a biological underpinning to the feeling of excessive,
intense inner emptiness, and you can see from the previous exercise how it
can be reinforced by being taught to fear not being busy and productive.
On the other hand, everyone feels bored, lonely, and disconnected from
the world sometimes. There is nothing at all unusual, wrong, or worri-
some about this affective state. The problem is the meaning that dysregulated eaters attach to not having anything to do: it is what causes them

to feel certain things — antsy, edgy, empty, frightened, stuck, paralyzed, adrift, or panicky.

■■ Get Smart!

What meaning do you ascribe to having nothing to do? What feelings arise from the meaning you make? Is your life really empty, or does it only feel that way? How does nonhunger eating make you feel better — and worse?

There is no brilliant, quick, one-size-fits-all answer for what to do when you feel inner emptiness or boredom. I could remind you that you have friends, and that there are activities you could do if you wanted to do them, both inside and outside your home. I could give you the standard advice of calling someone, getting out, or finding something interesting to engage your mind or body.

However, my instinct and clinical experience tell me that you will need to dig deeper (via self-reflection, talking with intimates, reading, or if these things don't help, getting professional help) to discover and address what's really bothering you. In fact, I'd wager that this is a must-do if you wish to improve your skills at balancing work and play and not turn to food when you're alone and bored. One book I recommend is *Dark Nights of the Soul: A Guide to Finding Your Way through Life's Ordeals* by Thomas Moore. Essentially, Moore advises readers to learn more about their "dark nights" — in this case your internal emptiness — as a way to understand what these moments are trying to teach them and what is needed so they can live their best possible lives.

Since We're into Serious Stuff, What's the Secret to Filling My Life with More Than Food?

The secret is that there is no secret, as in: if you come a little closer, I'll whisper it in your ear. What will fill up your life in a meaningful way is something only you can discover. Each of us is tasked with finding that out on our own. And as to secrets, there is no one thing that amounts to a foolproof plan for giving your life meaning. In the same way that there are many individuals who would be a good match for you, there are many avenues that will enrich your life and breathe passion and satisfaction into it.

Sadly, it's so easy to make existence seem meaningful through obsessing about food and weight — dieting, engaging in abusive eating, and making ourselves miserable afterward — that many troubled eaters never get to the root of their difficulties with emptiness and lack of fulfillment. Each of us has a path to take, and each of us has to stay on it until we find ourselves. Maybe you believe you'll be fulfilled only when you're engaged in activities that benefit humankind. But not everyone can be out there on the front lines like Doctors Without Borders, or do public service by running for city council, or advance science by discovering renewable energy sources or miracle vaccines. Maybe you believe that being adored by the public will give you what you crave, but think of all the writers, artists, actors, musicians, and celebrities with mental health or addiction problems.

Now consider some ordinary people you know who seem to love life and life seems to love them back. They're not running around trying to fill up the proverbial hole in their soul; but rather, life seems to burst from them because they're content with whatever they're doing. Some work outside the home and some inside; some care for their own children, and some care for other people's children; some are well known in their communities, and some pass through life preferring to be left alone to follow their own star. What I'm saying is that *there's no one way to feed an empty life*, and the only way to discover what will nourish you is by trial and error and listening to what calls your name.

I've been privy to a great deal of this kind of seeking since I moved to Sarasota, Florida, in 2005 and came to know many people who are retired or semiretired. Some newcomers like me have simply continued the same work they did wherever they last lived. In my case, that was providing therapy, doing tele-coaching, teaching, and writing. Others had had their fill of former careers and were looking for something new to engage or challenge them. Some found it right away, and some took a long time, while others are still searching.

I see the same dynamics in the twentysomethings I treat for eating disorders. Although many are on a career path, they still seem to be craning their necks and squinting their eyes looking ahead for fulfillment rather than enjoying what's available to them in the moment. These same undercurrents are there for empty nesters and for people who are recently divorced or widowed. Shifts in status like these often generate situational self-doubts and feelings of unfulfillment that generally pass with time.

But many dysregulated eaters appear to have lived with an inner void for most of their lives. If you are one of these people, be careful not to go overboard with activity just to feed the void, because the absence of bustling around is going to make natural downtime seem even emptier. Look inward and ask yourself what is missing, even as you are keeping your eyes and heart wide open for opportunities to make connections to other people and for activities that cement your connection to yourself.

▰▰ Get Smart!

Have you felt an inner void ever since you can remember, or is yours attributable to a change in status or venue? How have you tried to fill this void, other than with food or dieting? Think about the times you felt fulfilled, not through busy-ness or achievement, but through a sense of inner peace or passion in your core. How did you make that happen? How can you make it happen now?

Don't I Need Passion, Purpose, or Meaning to Feel Well Balanced in My Life?

To feel alive and emotionally engaged with the world and other people, it helps to have a reason to get up in the morning, but that reason need not be something special or unique. The problem with using words like *passion*, *purpose*, and *meaning* is that they sound grandiose and exceptional, as if you have to go through some spiritual awakening or to experience transcendence to find them for yourself. The fact is, some people do need an epiphany to awaken from their walking slumber and realize exactly what nourishes them. Other people seem to stumble upon such a thing, give up what they have for what they've stumbled upon, and never look back. Yet others leap from challenge to challenge, and this string of challenges ensures engagement throughout a lifetime.

You may find your passion, purpose, or meaning in work, especially if it involves creativity; yet there are many clever folks who feel truly inspired only by using their creativity for something larger than themselves. Maybe a choreographer begins an inner-city dance troupe or, as an artist friend of mine has done, becomes an adjunct professor at a community college. Alternatively, if you're in business or are a professional, that may not be where your juice comes from. I have a retired friend who, while in the middle of writing a book, resumed painting, something he hadn't done for decades. Now that's all he wants to do, and his manuscript probably will remain forever unfinished.

A client of mine, a businesswoman and mother of young adult children, makes jewelry and loses herself so entirely in her craft that she forgets to eat. Another client works in a city but drives out to an animal sanctuary in the country every weekend to learn how to engage with and care for wild birds. One friend is a movie buff, living and breathing everything cinema. A dentist I know plays in a rock-and-roll band, and a friend who's an insurance broker is working on reigniting a singing career. I know people who are news junkies and who come alive through reading and discussing politics, and a few folks who've been enthralled for years with developing their family trees. I have another friend who returned to school in her sixties to earn a social-work degree and then wrote a memoir.

What I'm trying to show you is that you can nourish yourself in an infinite number of ways. Of course, even when you're fulfilled by work or play most of the time, it doesn't mean you won't ever feel lonely or experience a kind of ennui, which sometimes settles over people. I went through a difficult period of ennui for about a year before I quit my methadone-clinic job, started my own psychotherapy practice, and began writing seriously. Loneliness and boredom are part of the human condition. They are certainly easier to ride through, however, when you know that they are temporary, that when you come through them you'll find or return to a more engaged, more impassioned life.

▪▪▪ Get Smart!

How have you sought passion, meaning, and purpose in life? How does eating prevent you from finding what you're looking for? The next time you feel bored, lonely, or unfulfilled and have the urge for food, what can you do or say to yourself rather than eat?

There Are So Many Things I Feel I Should Do; How Will I Ever Find the Time to Play?

Ah! Therein lies the rub — all those pushy "shoulds." If you ever want to find a balance between work and play, you would do well to give up commands like the S-word. Here's why. People who joyfully and fluidly keep their lives in balance don't run on words like *should*. To get where they want to go or be, they don't order or bully themselves around.

Tell me, when someone says you *should* or *shouldn't* do something, what's your reaction? When they insist you *need to be* or *must not be* a certain way, how does that make you feel? If you're like most people — me included — commands like these make you bristle and, worse, sometimes make you want to do exactly the opposite of what you're being instructed to do, even though you may not be aware of it.

Let's face it, by the time you're out of knee pants, you don't much want anyone telling you what to do. That doesn't mean they're wrong in doing so, or that you won't benefit from listening to what they have to say. It just means that these words kick up a good deal of dander within us because we associate them with childhood, when we heard — and had to heed — them 24/7. And because you had little or no choice in avoiding what your parents said you had to do back then, now when you hear commands, you often want to rebel. It's a natural instinct.

Think about words like *should, need to, have to, must, ought to,* and *are supposed to.* Or their opposites: *shouldn't, mustn't,* and *aren't supposed to.* They're called external motivators and don't work well in the long run. Here's why. Tell yourself, "I have to clean the bathroom," and notice the prickles of resentment or annoyance, the "Yeah, make me" attitude that can spring up from seemingly nowhere. If you frequently use these words to get yourself to do this and not do that, you'll more than likely rebel against them. The reason is that these were the words you heard constantly as a kid. If your parents regularly issued commands, rather than asked or encouraged you to take or not take action, you're probably sick to death of following orders; yet ironically, there you are, ordering yourself around without realizing it.

So ditch the self-directives. You're far better off using internal motivators like *want, would like, desire, wish*, or *prefer* to express intention. After all, you do want to clean the bathroom (because you'll feel good when it's done), you *wish* to take the car in to be fixed on your day off (so that it runs well in the future), you *prefer* to work overtime (in order to worry less about making ends meet), you *desire* to take care of your sick child and pass on those free movie tickets (because you'll feel proud of your parenting skills), and you *would like* to have dinner with your husband's crabby parents (because he does things he doesn't want to do in order to make you happy). You don't *need* to do any of those things. The only thing we need to do in this life is die; everything else — you make a choice and live with the consequence — is optional.

This concept can be a tough sell to dysregulated eaters. They'll argue with me that they *should* eat healthfully, *must* stop overeating, *need to* lose weight, are *supposed to* be productive, *have to* take good care of themselves, and *ought to* exercise. And I'll answer right back that they need not do any of these things as long as they're willing to live with the results of not doing them. Eventually, most people start to see the light.

All we ever have is desires, which, by their very nature, often compete with other desires. For instance, I want to stop writing now because I'm getting tired, and I also want to complete this chapter tonight. It's not that I *should* or *need* to finish it. I really want to — and I really don't. Can you see the benefits of using internal motivators? When you do, you're weighing words of equal value against each other, and they can have a fair fight. Commands simply are fraught with too much negative baggage to be useful in decision making.

"And what," you might ask, "does this have to do with balancing work and play?" Everything, absolutely everything. When you command yourself to work, do chores, or take actions using external motivators, your natural response is to balk, rebel, and not do them. It's as simple as that. Using those words is a setup for ensuring that you won't do what you keep telling yourself you "ought" to do. *Capisce?*

That's one of the reasons you have such difficulty working when it's time to work and playing when it's time to play. When you're working, you would like to be playing because you hardly ever give yourself that kind of break; and, even when you do, you feel so guilty that you don't enjoy yourself. When you're playing, you're convinced you should be working; and that takes all the joy and pleasure out of it. And all this nonsense starts with words like *should* and *need to* or their negatives. The way out of this bind is to — duh — stop using these words. If you want to work and you also want to take a break from work, well, that seems reasonable. Hash it out with yourself. Don't bully yourself into deciding you *need* to do something you *don't* need to do and, in the process, set the stage for instant rebellion.

It helps to think of using words like *need* and *have to* as a finger poking you in the back, telling you to move along. Who would ever want that? On the other hand, words like *want* and *desire* are more like a finger inside that beckons you forward. It's clear which is the better motivator, isn't it?

Moreover, when you feel you *ought to* be working and won't allow yourself a break, how do you oh-so-cleverly manage to take one after all? You don't even need three guesses to answer that. You make sure you cut loose by eating, even if you're not the least bit hungry, even if you're stuffed to the gills. Paradoxically, when you rebel against yourself — for who else are you, as a fully autonomous adult, rebelling against? — you do it in the form of abusing food and your body. It may sound strange, but it's true.

▓▓ Get Smart!

Do you often bully yourself with external motivators like *should* and *have to*, *shouldn't* and *mustn't*? Are you willing to swap them for internal motivators like *want* and *wish*? In your own words, describe how you rebel against doing things you don't want to do by abusing food.

To sum up, there are several skills to learn regarding balancing work and play:

- Comb through your beliefs and make sure they're not lop-sided — heavily prowork and pro-productivity, or heavily proplay — and that they support a sensible balance between the two.
- Make sure you understand exactly what play is, and that you're not doing it with a hidden agenda to get something done.
- Explore and understand your "need" for busy-ness and productivity.
- Fully examine the issue of perceiving your life as empty and trying to feed that void with food. Take time to decide what might bring passion, meaning, and purpose to your life, but don't even think of pushing yourself into or toward anything. You'll know when you find it, and you'll benefit from giving things a chance to engage you.
- Stop bullying yourself with external motivators that make you likely to rebel and abuse food, and start using internal motivators.
- We hear so much talk these days about mindfulness, but remember, please, that there's a time to be mindful and a time to be mindless.

Over time, you'll develop the skill to keep work and play in balance — and you'll find that unwanted eating is less of a problem.

Skill Boosters

1. Define play according to how you understand it.
2. What three words come to mind to describe how you feel about work and daily-living tasks?
3. What three words come to mind to describe how you feel about play or relaxation?
4. Recall an anecdote that nails down exactly how your family

felt or feels about anyone not doing their job or not doing it well.

5. Recall an anecdote that shows how you absorbed your family's message about hard work and productivity or rebelled against it.

6. What play activities do you wish you'd done more of as a child or adolescent?

7. Recall the best times you had at play as a child or adolescent.

8. Read your reframed beliefs about work and play aloud three times a day in front of a mirror, as well as first thing when you awaken and last thing before you go to sleep.

9. During the day, check in with yourself when you're working or playing and see how you're feeling, especially if you're working and desire a break or are playing and are ready to get back to work.

10. Practice sitting while doing nothing for one minute for three days, three minutes for three days, five minutes for three days, and so forth, until you've worked yourself into comfortably sitting and doing nothing for ten minutes a day. (And notice that the world doesn't end!)

11. Whenever you have the urge to eat at work when you're not hungry, recognize it as a desire to take a break; and know that it's about downtime, not chow time.

12. Ask people close to you to point out when you use external motivators, and try to catch yourself using them. Then replace them with internal motivators.

13. When you play or relax, shoo away guilty thoughts.

14. Consider effective ways to deal with people who might have a difficult time seeing you spend more time at play or relaxing.

15. To find out what excites you and what bores you to tears, notice how engaged or unengaged you are in your activities throughout the day. Do more of what excites you and less of what bores you.

16. Review your day, each day, to assess whether your work and play felt balanced and what adjustments you might have made to enjoy a better balance.

After completing the Life Skills Postassessment, you'll reach chapter 10, which will pull all the threads in this book together for you.

Life Skills Postassessment

It's time to do your postassessment, which I've tucked between the pre-ceding chapters on individual skill sets and the final chapter on integrating these skills into your life. Take a few deep breaths and make sure you're wearing your curiosity cap and not your Wicked Witch of the West hat. This questionnaire is designed to help you determine what you've learned and which specific, challenging skill sets need more attention. No judging yourself, pretty please, if you're not as competent in a skill area as you'd like to be. Instead of being hard on yourself, practice curiosity and com-passion and maintain the growth-oriented mind-set discussed earlier: rec-ognize that, with practice, you'll feel a good deal better about your skills as time goes on.

Remember that there are no right or wrong responses to the statements in this questionnaire, and give each one some thought before answering as honestly as you can. This is not a final exam. In fact, I encourage you to run through this assessment again one month, three months, six months, and a year from now. You'll be surprised at how quickly you acquire skills when you put your mind to it.

Instructions: Circle the number that best describes your response to each statement, with the number 1 representing *least true* and 10 representing *most true*.

1. Overall, I have effective life skills.

   1   2   3   4   5   6   7   8   9   10

2. I surround myself with people who have effective life skills.

   1   2   3   4   5   6   7   8   9   10

3. Improved life skills would help me eat "normally" and attain and maintain a healthy weight.

   1   2   3   4   5   6   7   8   9   10

4. I take excellent care of my health.

   1   2   3   4   5   6   7   8   9   10

5. I have routine medical tests, follow doctors' orders, and take care of emergency medical concerns right away.

1   2   3   4   5   6   7   8   9   10

6. I get sufficient sleep most nights.

1   2   3   4   5   6   7   8   9   10

7. I take vitamins and supplements or medication consistently.

1   2   3   4   5   6   7   8   9   10

8. I get exercise (formal or informal) on a regular basis.

1   2   3   4   5   6   7   8   9   10

9. I am generally in touch with and can identify my feelings.

1   2   3   4   5   6   7   8   9   10

10. I value and am willing to experience all my feelings.

1   2   3   4   5   6   7   8   9   10

11. Rather than judging them, I am curious about my feelings.

1   2   3   4   5   6   7   8   9   10

12. I can tolerate intense and uncomfortable or conflicting feelings.

1   2   3   4   5   6   7   8   9   10

13. I express emotions appropriately and effectively.

1   2   3   4   5   6   7   8   9   10

14. I comfort and calm myself effectively.

1   2   3   4   5   6   7   8   9   10

15. For the most part, I live consciously and in the present.

1   2   3   4   5   6   7   8   9   10

16. I don't spend time unnecessarily worrying about the past.

1   2   3   4   5   6   7   8   9   10

17. I don't spend time unnecessarily worrying about the future.

1   2   3   4   5   6   7   8   9   10

18. I know that whatever befalls me in life, I will manage.

   1   2   3   4   5   6   7   8   9   10

19. I plan for the future, then let it take care of itself.

   1   2   3   4   5   6   7   8   9   10

20. I am comfortable in most social situations.

   1   2   3   4   5   6   7   8   9   10

21. I am generally honest and share my feelings with intimates.

   1   2   3   4   5   6   7   8   9   10

22. Intimates care about me as much as I care about them.

   1   2   3   4   5   6   7   8   9   10

23. I set boundaries with intimates, and they respect them.

   1   2   3   4   5   6   7   8   9   10

24. I take care of myself as well as I take care of others.

   1   2   3   4   5   6   7   8   9   10

25. I'm good at knowing who to trust and who not to trust.

   1   2   3   4   5   6   7   8   9   10

26. I know how to make and keep wonderful friends.

   1   2   3   4   5   6   7   8   9   10

27. I'm pretty even emotionally and avoid emotional extremes.

   1   2   3   4   5   6   7   8   9   10

28. I generally know when enough is enough.

   1   2   3   4   5   6   7   8   9   10

29. I don't tend to frequently overdo or underdo.

   1   2   3   4   5   6   7   8   9   10

30. I don't depend on others to regulate me emotionally.

   1   2   3   4   5   6   7   8   9   10

31. When I'm with difficult people, I stay on an even keel.

   1   2   3   4   5   6   7   8   9   10

32. I don't think in all-or-nothing, black-or-white terms.

    1   2   3   4   5   6   7   8   9   10

33. I value both structure and freedom.

    1   2   3   4   5   6   7   8   9   10

34. I'm skilled at troubleshooting and problem solving.

    1   2   3   4   5   6   7   8   9   10

35. I'm neither too cautious nor impulsive in decision making.

    1   2   3   4   5   6   7   8   9   10

36. I don't second-guess myself after making a decision.

    1   2   3   4   5   6   7   8   9   10

37. I don't put off decisions because they're hard to make.

    1   2   3   4   5   6   7   8   9   10

38. I have confidence in my critical-thinking skills.

    1   2   3   4   5   6   7   8   9   10

39. I generally reach my goals.

    1   2   3   4   5   6   7   8   9   10

40. I'm good at creating concrete, realistic goals for myself.

    1   2   3   4   5   6   7   8   9   10

41. I know how to divide big goals into smaller ones.

    1   2   3   4   5   6   7   8   9   10

42. I'm skilled at sustaining the effort needed to reach my goals.

    1   2   3   4   5   6   7   8   9   10

43. I'm good at maintaining my hard-won achievements.

    1   2   3   4   5   6   7   8   9   10

44. I don't sabotage my progress or achievements.

    1   2   3   4   5   6   7   8   9   10

45. I recognize that all progress consists of baby steps.

    1   2   3   4   5   6   7   8   9   10

46. My goals are composed of my wants, not "shoulds."

    1   2   3   4   5   6   7   8   9   10

47. I can easily ask for or accept help in reaching my goals.

    1   2   3   4   5   6   7   8   9   10

48. I always speak kindly to myself about myself.

    1   2   3   4   5   6   7   8   9   10

49. I don't let other people be unkind or hurtful to me.

    1   2   3   4   5   6   7   8   9   10

50. I don't have to be perfect.

    1   2   3   4   5   6   7   8   9   10

51. I value myself and expect others to value me too.

    1   2   3   4   5   6   7   8   9   10

52. I both love myself unconditionally and strive to do better.

    1   2   3   4   5   6   7   8   9   10

53. I'm generally more curious about, than critical of, my mistakes.

    1   2   3   4   5   6   7   8   9   10

54. I take failure in stride and learn from it.

    1   2   3   4   5   6   7   8   9   10

55. I have a stable sense of myself.

    1   2   3   4   5   6   7   8   9   10

56. I live a life balanced between obligations and play.

    1   2   3   4   5   6   7   8   9   10

57. I can relax and let go fairly easily in healthy ways.

    1   2   3   4   5   6   7   8   9   10

58. I know when I'm ready to work or play or relax.

    1   2   3   4   5   6   7   8   9   10

59. I rarely procrastinate or rebel against commitments.

    1   2   3   4   5   6   7   8   9   10

60. I live purposely and know the meaning of my life.

    1   2   3   4   5   6   7   8   9   10

Okay, have you recovered from doing your postassessment? Please, if you're a perfectionist, listen up. Now that you've done your assessing and approach the final chapter of this book, I hope you're not expecting to be proficient in all the life skills you've been reading about. I assume that, like the rest of us muddling along on this planet, you've been working on improving at least some of these skills for quite a while, and that this book has given you the encouragement and guidance to keep on improving them.

CHAPTER 10

Integrating Life Skills into Eating "Normally"

I Get It — Gain the Life Skills, Lose the Food Problem!

We all need essential life skills for health, happiness, and well-being. In addition, you happen to need them in order to end your eating problems. Perhaps you're even saying to yourself right now, "Gee, maybe my problems were never really about food in the first place, but instead were the result of not having effective life skills." I wouldn't have written *Outsmarting Overeating* if I'd thought otherwise!

Now that you're almost finished with this book, the question is how to move forward. My fervent wish is that you will use compassion, pace yourself, view difficult experiences with food and other disappointments as learning experiences, and avoid trying to be perfect at anything except being imperfect. Remember, the goal of life is not to be flawless but to take in all it has to offer and live each day to its fullest. Isn't that a lot easier than always pushing yourself to go for the gold? I guarantee that you'll do better at some skill sets than others, and that life will sorely test your abilities with all of them. That's been my experience; and when you think of it, how could it be otherwise?

Now it's time to consider how to apply the skill sets you've been learning and to improve your relationship with food. I've talked a bit about eating in each chapter, but intentionally less than you may have hoped, because I wanted you to put your full attention on skills, not on your perceived feeding failures. The truth is, getting troubled eaters to focus on their eating is as easy as pie. But it's heavy lifting to get them to shift gears and put attention on other aspects of their lives that aren't going so swimmingly. And now it's time to combine the two.

So, let's put some of those skills — say, the skills for living consciously and staying regulated — to work right away. Now that you've done the postassessment, what are you thinking and feeling? Be sure to stay in the present rather than drifting toward thoughts about how you've done with food in the past or jumping ahead to how you might manage it better in the future. Anchor yourself to current pinpoints of thought and emotion, and see where they take you as you express compassion for, rather than judgment about, yourself.

If you start to feel upset that you're not where you want to be, simply note that your response to the assessment triggered some emotional dysregulation. Change your thinking and come back to a centered, neutral position, take a few deep breaths, and use positive self-talk to reregulate yourself. If you want to handle, by yourself, what's come up, dig deep for your inner strengths. If not, could you share your feelings with someone, write about them in a journal, or post your distress on a message board?

In terms of problem solving and using critical-thinking skills, consider what you're feeling. What can you do right now to feel more encouraged and hopeful? If you have ideas in mind, write them down. Use your critical-thinking skills to test your feelings against rational thinking and your experience. For example, if you feel like eating because you're bummed that you haven't made the progress you hoped to make, ask yourself if food will truly help. Make a list of how you want to spend the rest of the day foodwise and otherwise. Tap into your wisest self. Because you've worked hard reading this book, go ahead and engage in something fun that will allow you to lose yourself and not have to use your brain to think or reflect.

How Do I Put These New Skills
I'm Learning into Action in Real Life?

Consider how you felt learning a new job. Every day was full of challenges, and perhaps you often felt that you weren't picking up skills and information as quickly as you wished. Now think about having learned that job and how you felt about it six months or a year or more later. You could probably do some of it in your sleep by now. Remember that you've chosen, or been thrown into, many situations — work, kids, taking care of aging or ill loved ones — in which you had to acquire skills on the proverbial job.

And you did it. Skill-building for better eating is no different. What you want to avoid is focusing on how poorly you did in the past, especially on your "mistakes." Make your mantra: "That was then, and this is now." And don't keep worrying about how you're going to do. The worry takes you away from the present, which is *the only place where learning and change can occur.* You can learn from the past and apply that wisdom to the future, but the actual, hard-core doing-things-differently can happen only in the moment. You can think about having done something, and about what will be done, but the only time you actually can *do* is in the here and now.

That noted, let me say that replaying an eating situation by purposefully spinning out your story with a different ending can be helpful. So, it's okay to consciously rerun the past and change your actions to give yourself a happier ending to an eating story. You also may find it valuable to spend time visualizing — called rehearsing — how you want to respond to difficult future situations in order to eat "normally." Notice that the life skill used in both situations is "living consciously." Your mind isn't drifting into the past without your awareness and making you feel hopeless, and it isn't anxiously rushing ahead trying to make the future turn out right for you. Rather, you're intentionally replaying a memory to analyze how you could have made a situation come out more successfully by using problem-solving and critical-thinking skills. Ditto when you're rehearsing: you're not unconsciously loading yourself up with pressure to do better but are intentionally imagining a future circumstance in order to plan out how you want to respond to it.

I've come up with a set of essential questions to ask yourself that will help you integrate into the real world the eight life skills discussed in this book. This protocol is similar to any ritual you follow. For example, when you want to drive, you automatically unlock your car and start up your engine, and maybe you shove in a CD or turn on the radio. As you start to pick up speed, you may even set your car on cruise control. Similarly, you follow a set of actions you barely think about when you reenter your house after vacation, are diapering your infant, or have to reset anything electrical in your house when the electricity goes out. Every time I leave the house, I unconsciously run through a list: Did I take my purse (because I have on more than one occasion caught myself halfway to somewhere without it)? Do I have my cell phone and sunglasses? Can I get a sighting of the cat so I know I haven't unintentionally closed her in a room? Are all the windows shut so I can set the house alarm? Think of a ritual or protocol that you engage in daily or weekly, one that is second nature by now, so that you barely notice going through it.

Following are the questions you'll want to get in the habit of asking yourself in order to integrate life skills into your world, with a special focus on those that will guide you toward "normal" eating. You can apply this eight-step protocol to any situation, whether it's one that happens down the road or one that is in your face right now. And don't worry, I'm going to take you through a whole bunch of examples to help you see how the questions are applicable and useful. Remember, it's all about enhancing your life skills!

1. Wellness and Physical Self-Care: How will this situation, advice, request, demand, interaction, occasion, or other circumstance affect my health and ability to take good care of myself physically, especially regarding eating?

2. Handling Emotions: How will I manage my emotions effectively in this situation or interaction or on this occasion?

3. Living Consciously: Rather than react automatically, how will I make conscious choices in this situation, interaction, or occasion or respond to this advice, request, or demand?

4. Building and Maintaining Relationships: How can I respond appropriately to this situation, advice, request, demand, interaction, or occasion in a way that honors myself and others?

5. Self-Regulation: What steps will I take to remain emotionally self-regulated regarding this situation, advice, request, demand, interaction, or occasion?

6. Problem Solving and Critical Thinking: How will I respond

to this situation, advice, request, demand, interaction, or occasion in a way that is based on effective problem solving and critical thinking?

7. Setting and Reaching Goals: What are my goals regarding this situation, advice, request, demand, interaction, or occasion, and what steps will I use to reach them?

8. Balancing Work and Play: How can I respond to this situation, advice, request, demand, interaction, or occasion in a way that maintains a balance between work and play?

Now that you know the questions, it's time to try some hypothetical scenarios and practice using this eight-step protocol. I'll start you off with my ideas for how you might think through your responses, then I'll let you try the rest on your own. Notice that I'm not going to make decisions for you, that I will only show you how you might make effective choices for yourself. Moreover, there are no right answers, and that's an important caveat. There are numerous ways to respond to each scenario. The point is to get you skilled in thinking about how to make effective choices, not how to find the right choice, because often there is no right choice, just one that is better or worse for you. Okay, here goes.

Scenario 1: It's Friday near closing time at work, and your boss asks you to stay late. All day you've been sensing that you're coming down with a cold, and you have tentative plans to attend a movie with a friend but nothing else scheduled for the weekend. Your boss rarely asks for anything at the last minute, but seems anxious to clear out her in-basket. What do you do?

According to the protocol, you would ask yourself:

1. Wellness and Physical Self-Care: How might staying late affect my impending cold? Might I avoid letting it become full blown by leaving on time and chilling out for the evening, even canceling the movie with my friend? Alternatively, might I work late and rest up over the weekend? If I stay, will I arrive home hungry and be more tempted to eat quickly or choose nonnutritious food; or can I run out and grab something now that will tide me over until I get home? How am I going to take care of feeding myself?

2. Handling Emotions: How will I feel emotionally if I work late or leave on time? Will I feel taken advantage of and resentful because my boss has sprung a last-minute demand on me? Will I feel guilty if I refuse her request and leave for home on time? Will my feelings be so out of control either way that they'll drive me to eat?

3. Living Consciously: Am I staying in the present while making this decision, or is my mind slipping backward, to a memory of my old boss who blew up at me when I refused to cancel my vacation and fill in for an employee who quit? Am I getting ahead of myself by focusing on a rumor that the company might be downsizing, and by worrying that a refusal of my boss's request might be a reason to can me?

4. Building and Maintaining Relationships: How will refusing my boss's request affect our relationship? If it will cause friction between us, is it still worth saying no? If I cancel going to the movie, how will that affect my friendship? Will my friend understand or be upset with me for backing out at the last minute? How will I handle her upset?

5. Self-Regulation: How has my boss's request affected my ability to self-regulate emotionally? Is it triggering memories of how my demanding father used to insist I stop playing and finish my chores? Am I getting so angry at my boss that I can't think straight? Whatever I decide, how will I feel better emotionally without turning to food?

6. Problem Solving and Critical Thinking: Is there evidence that my boss's request is or might become part of a pattern of asking me to work late frequently? Is there a way to create a win-win situation here? What are my options? Stay late and cancel my outing with my friend or meet her for a late movie? Leave on time and take work home? Leave on time and come in over the weekend to finish up? Any other options?

7. Setting and Reaching Goals: What are my goals with this job: Staying with it over the long term and moving up the ladder? Or do I plan on leaving soon, so that tonight's decision

doesn't mean a great deal to my career? Will saying no affect my job security?

8. Balancing Work and Play: Is there a way to respond so I'll feel that work and play are in balance? Maybe stay late at work and do nothing else over the weekend? Maybe go home and come back tomorrow? Do I want to forgo the pleasure of seeing a movie with my friend, after working hard all week, to spend more time on the job?

How'd that go? Is that how you would have sussed out the situation? Or would you have panicked and said yes without thinking things through or declined immediately because you hate it when people just assume you'll do what they ask or pressure you to do things? Even though it looks as if you might need to spend a great deal of time running through this protocol, these eight quick steps will get you in the habit of thoroughly analyzing your response options until your skills automatically become razor sharp and kick right in.

Let's try a couple more scenarios.

Scenario 2: You're remarried and your spouse's kids from a first marriage are coming to stay with you and your three kids over the holidays. Your spouse didn't exactly ask you first, but you know how much it means for him or her to have parent-child time together, so you didn't make a fuss when you weren't told that the kids decided to take an earlier flight than you'd expected. Holidays are always a busy time, and you like to make everything as perfect as possible for everyone. That's how you function in holiday mode, and you're usually exhausted and about five pounds heavier by the end of the year.

1. Wellness and Physical Self-Care: How will I take care of myself physically with so much going on and so many people to care for? When can I block out time on the calendar to exercise and be active? What strategies can I develop to manage food so that I make healthy choices, and where can I post a list of eating guidelines for myself so that I will read them over often? How can I find time every day to be alone, unwind, and care for my body and mind? How will I ensure that I get enough sleep every night no matter what's going

on? Who must I talk with beforehand to make sure my self-care plans are clear and firmly in place? How will I approach my family about them?

2. Handling Emotions: How do I really feel about my spouse's kids coming to visit? How do I feel about not being asked? Do I have leftover anger or resentment? Would I have said yes or no if asked? How am I feeling about spending time with my stepchildren? Do I want to eat to lessen the intensity of my feelings? What will I do if I start to feel out of control emotionally? What's my plan to keep myself from abusing food?

3. Living Consciously: How can I not drive myself crazy anxious about making things just right? How will I remind myself to stay in the moment and not try to micromanage everyone's time? How will I make sure to have some fun myself over the holidays without turning to food for it? What steps will help me eat mindfully at every meal?

4. Building and Maintaining Relationships: What can I do to help my spouse's kids and our kids have a good time separately and together? How will having stepkids here affect my relationship with my own children? Will I promise to be honest with my spouse about how things are going, or will I say that things are fine when they're not? Will I request beforehand that my spouse be the one to take special care of his or her kids and not dump all responsibility on me?

5. Self-Regulation: How will being thrown off my usual routine affect me? If ever there were a time for me to abuse food, this would be it, when I'll be feeling so discombobulated, so how can I stay centered? What, other than food, will help me reregulate myself when I'm knocked off course emotionally, which is likely to happen no matter how well I plan?

6. Problem Solving and Critical Thinking: Are there any problems in making arrangements that need to be taken care of ahead of time? Who will help me? Might it be a good idea to talk with my spouse ASAP and divvy up tasks as well as

arrange some preplanned activities? Would it be a good idea for my spouse and me to have time each day to check in with each other to assess how things are going between us and with the kids? In what ways have I avoided overeating during previous holidays, or in other family situations, that I can apply to this situation this year? How have I fallen into nonhunger or mindless eating during past holidays, and what steps can I take to do better this year?

7. Setting and Reaching Goals: What are my goals for this holiday — to be the world's greatest spouse, parent, stepparent, or host or hostess? To make sure I don't abuse food? To enjoy myself? To get through the holidays without losing my mind?

8. Balancing Work and Play: How can I make sure I get done what I need to and still have sufficient time to relax? What will my spouse and both sets of children need to do so that everything doesn't rest on my shoulders? How will I make it clear to everyone that I will take time for myself whether it pleases them or not? How will I follow through with my plan to take play or alone time even if it bothers or inconveniences others?

Perhaps you see how this scenario is more complicated than the last one and requires putting greater skill into action. There's a good deal more going on that might precipitate opportunities for stress eating, and as a result there's an increased need to focus on yourself. If you practice life skills every chance you get, you can't help but exponentially elevate the likelihood that they'll emerge naturally when the pressure's on. Can you see how honing your life skills would make even the previous scenario a great deal easier on you and your appetite?

Okay, let's run through one final scenario together.

Scenario 3: You and a bunch of your old high school friends think it would be fun to get away together for a three-night cruise. You're still crazy about two of them, one you can take or leave, and the other is a riot to hang with but a spoilsport unless she gets her way. The last time you were together, she went from ignoring you to relentlessly picking on you in her hey-I'm-just-teasing way. Plus, you're terrified that all that yummy cruise food and the hyperfocus on eating will put too much stress on your desire to eat "normally" when most of your friends have crummy food habits. You sorely need a vacation, and this cruise has ports you're dying to visit, but you're really torn about whether to go.

1. Wellness and Physical Self-Care: How will this trip enhance or impair my health? If I intend to eat "normally," what will I have to think, feel, and do every day for that to happen? Do I tend to get seasick? How will my friends' careless eating habits affect me, and will my best intentions get steamrolled by groupthink?

2. Handling Emotions: If I'm already anxious about the trip, how am I going to feel while on it? How can I ignore my friend if she acts up and yet still have a good time? How much of my reaction to her is triggered by her resemblance to my bossy older sister, who used to tease me and make jokes at my expense? What attitude do I want to have in order to be emotionally mature on the trip? Will I get so upset that I abuse food to handle my emotions?

3. Living Consciously: Will I worry the whole time I'm away that I'm not going to enjoy myself or that I'll eat crazily? Even if things are fine with that one friend, will I be on edge while waiting for her to zap me? How will I eat mindfully at every meal? How can I stay present at every moment of the trip so that I enjoy myself?

4. Building and Maintaining Relationships: How can I use my positive friendships to buffer my relationship with the one friend I don't care for so much? If I don't go on the cruise, will it upset my friends or will they be relieved? Will they invite me on a group outing again? Will my forgoing the trip ruin individual relationships with my friends?

5. Self-Regulation: Will my friends want to do everything together as a group, or will I have time to myself? How will I let them know how important self-time is to me? How will I follow through on my plan to go off on my own if need be,

even if it angers or disappoints my friends? What will I do to reregulate myself, other than eat, if I feel pressured or upset?

6. Problem Solving and Critical Thinking: What are the pros and cons of going? Is there any other available info about the trip that would help me make a decision? How might considering my previous experience with these friends help me decide? Who can I talk with to help me decide? Am I in denial about any factors that I would like to pay attention to? Is it wishful thinking to believe that I can go on the cruise and eat "normally," or is there evidence that this is highly unlikely?

7. Setting and Reaching Goals: What are my goals for the trip — to hang out with friends, sightsee, get away from work and routine, or have adventures? When will my friends and I talk about our goals for the trip to make sure they mesh? Do I want to make it a goal to eat "normally" while on the cruise, or just give myself a vacation from thinking about everything I put in my mouth? What goals will help me stay active on the cruise?

8. Balancing Work and Play: Is the timing right to take a vacation, and is this cruise the right activity? Would I be better off passing on the invitation and planning another getaway more to my liking, or will I regret missing this cruise and having fun with my friends?

Are you getting the hang of it? It's easy to apply life skills to any problem, although not every situation will need all your skills. You get to pick and choose, and after a while you'll know which ones are required. Mainly, what using life skills does is slow down the process of automatically reacting to what's going on inside of and around you. It helps you identify your emotions but not rely on them for decision making. It takes you off Fantasy Island, especially in response to food, exercise, and self-care, and firmly plants your feet on this earth. It brings many of the same abilities you use at work into your personal life: evaluating pros and cons, taking history into account, and choosing options based on rationality and not your whim of the moment.

To give yourself practice employing your newly acquired life skills in the eating arena, use the eight-point protocol to consider what to do under the following circumstances:

- Scenario: For years, your mother, now ninety, made twenty kinds of Christmas cookies and stored them in the freezer for holiday gifts and gatherings. Recently, your sister-in-law had the idea of making a "recipe book of Mom's cookies," insisting that everyone in the family bake a few kinds, take pictures of them for a book for Mom, and keep them frozen until the holidays. You've been learning to be a "normal" eater and practicing life skills for about six months, and you aren't sure how you feel about making and storing the holiday cookies for the recipe book. Having all these delicacies around might be too tempting for you at this stage of learning to eat "normally."

- Scenario: Your younger brother just lost his job and wants to move in with you "for just a little while." Last time he did this, he failed to clean up after himself and ate a constant diet of junk food no matter what you cooked for him. Because you live alone, it is completely your decision whether you deny or accede to his request; but you're not sure what to do, mostly because your brother has pulled you out of several jams and you want to return the favor. Also, recently he seems to be making better decisions and finally maturing. You've just started reading books on "normal" eating and are intrigued by the idea of learning how to eat healthfully, and you wonder if his living with you might derail your plans.

- Scenario: Your entire office is starting a diet contest, to be accompanied by a weekly weigh-in. You've gained and lost hundreds of pounds, and dieting is the last thing you want to do, although you're unhappy with your current weight. The office manager is asking staff to choose up teams. Everyone seems gung ho. You don't want to be the odd person out, but you worry that dieting will trigger binge eating as it always has in the past. Plus, you're trying not to weigh yourself, because you'd rather focus exclusively on trying to eat well without the pressure of the scale.

- Scenario: Your mother has been nagging you to join her Saturday morning walking club. You enjoy the men and women in it, you could use structured exercise, and Saturday morning is a perfect time for you. But you haven't gotten along well with your mother since you were young enough to sit on her lap, and you don't want to make the relationship more strained than it already is. You can't decide whether to join the walking club.

- Scenario: You've been noticing that your aunt, who lives with her brother, your widowed father, is getting more forgetful. She's like a second mother to you because, when you were a child, your mother was sick a great deal of the time and your aunt moved in with your family to help raise you while your father worked. When you were old enough, she moved out, and you took care of your mother and moved out only after she died. Although Dad refuses to get his sister checked out medically, you believe she has Alzheimer's. Dad wants you to move in with them when your apartment lease is up — you can have your old room back — and you're not sure what to do. You've been enjoying taking care of just little old you — eating healthfully and exercising — for the first time in your life, but you feel the call of duty. You're afraid that having more people to care for will make it difficult to care for yourself.

- Scenario: You have what feels like a once-in-a-lifetime opportunity, a scholarship to study abroad. Your parents and college professors and adviser are all for it, but you're scared of being off on your own and you fear how a new environment will influence your relationship with food. Eating goes best for you when you're alone in your studio apartment and have control over what you buy, cook, and eat. You're fearful of being in a new place with new foods, so you're thinking of turning down the scholarship.

How did you do while using your new life skills in these hypothetical situations? Are you getting the knack of running through the protocol more quickly and adeptly? What I'd like you to pay attention to is whether you had previously used these skills in decision making, and what you learned from doing so in these scenarios that you can apply in your life. After all, it's not that hard to decide what's best for an imaginary person. But as you acquire life skills, you'll find it easier and easier to keep them at the ready for the real world you live in.

Here's one other way you can practice life skills without any consequence to you. Every time you hear of a problem situation — just listen to friends, coworkers, and family, and you'll hear plenty of them — use the eight-point protocol to consider how you would suss things out. Consider what emotions you'd have. Maybe they'd be the same as someone else's, but maybe not. Think about how you would stay rational and present while resolving whatever is troublesome rather than reactively jumping to a decision. Take time to come up with a solution that reflects most, if not all, of the eight-point protocol. Notice if others use similar strategies or simply dive into solutions headfirst without engaging in much rational thinking. If you continue to imagine how you'd solve other people's problems, similar problems will be a great deal easier when they're your own.

Well, here we are at the end of the book. But for you, I hope, it's not an ending but a beginning. My wish is that your growing competencies open up a brand-new chapter in your life, one that is skill filled, more satisfying and pleasurable, and that your new abilities keep moving you along toward "normal" eating. I promise that, as you slowly acquire new skills, your self-care will improve exponentially. Everything will come together in good time.

Acknowledgments

Many thanks to Georgia Hughes, New World Library's editorial director, and to the rest of the editorial staff for their gentle guidance and expertise. And oodles of gratitude to Janice M. Pieroni, Esq., my literary agent and friend, who is always a pleasure to work with, from shaping up my manuscript to finding it a happy home.

Notes

Introduction

3 *"abilities for adaptive and positive behaviour"*: Skills for Health, World Health Organization's Information Series on School Health, Document 9 (Geneva: WHO, 2003), p. 8, www.who.int/school_youth_health/media/en/sch_skills 4health_03.pdf, accessed July 27, 2014.

4 *"You did the best that you knew how"*: Maya Angelou, Maya Angelou Quotes website, www.mayaangelouquotes.org/page/4/, accessed July 19, 2014.

Chapter 1. The Definition and Purpose of Life Skills

12 *five basic life skills that span every culture*: World Health Organization, Mental Health Promotion, Partners in Life Skills Education, "Conclusions from a United Nations Inter-Agency Meeting," Geneva, 1999, five basic life skills that are relevant across cultures, www.who.int/mental_health/media/en/30.pdf, accessed August 14, 2014.

19 *ten thousand hours is the average number of hours*: Malcolm Gladwell, *Outliers: The Story of Success* (New York: Little, Brown, 2007), 39.

24 *"sophisticated methods of assessing beliefs, opinions"*: Ronald J. Massey, "Glossary of Common Psychological Terms," s.v. "Critical Thinking Skills," Ronald J. Massey, PhD, and Associates website, accessed July 27, 2014, www.drronmassey.com /Glossary.html.

Chapter 3. Handling Emotions

47 *"In my view, if you forget everything else"*: Robert E. Thayer, *Calm Energy: How People Regulate Mood with Food and Exercise* (New York: Oxford University Press, 2001), 8.

48 *"less than 90 seconds"*: Jill Bolte Taylor, *My Stroke of Insight: A Brain Scientist's Personal Journey* (New York: Viking, 2006), 146.

56 *Most of the time when we're reacting strongly* : Jon Connelly, PhD, LCSW, "Clinical Hypnosis with Rapid Trauma Resolution," clinical training manual (revised March 16, 2010), 37.

59 *"emotional intelligence"*: Daniel Goleman, *Emotional Intelligence: Why It Can Matter More Than IQ* (New York: Bantam, 1995).

Chapter 4. Living Consciously

70 *how little attention we pay to everyday life*: Thomas Moore, *Care of the Soul: A Guide for Cultivating Depth and Sacredness in Everyday Life* (New York: HarperCollins, 1992).

Chapter 7. Problem Solving and Critical Thinking

126 *"has three central concerns: positive emotions"*: "Frequently Asked Questions," Positive Psychology Center, University of Pennsylvania, www.ppc.sas.upenn.edu /faqs.htm, accessed August 8, 2013.

135 *Attributes of critical thinkers*: Emily R. Lai, *Critical Thinking: A Literature Review*, June 2011, Pearson Assessments, www.pearsonassessments.com/hai/images/tmrs /criticalthinkingreviewfinal.pdf.

135 *"capable of taking a position or changing a position"*: Robert H. Ennis quoted in "Overview of Critical Thinking Skills," American Dental Education Association, accessed August 27, 2013, www.adea.org/adeacci/Resources/Critical-Thinking -Skills-Toolkit/Pages/Overview-of-Critical-Thinking-Skills.aspx.

Chapter 8. Setting and Reaching Goals

142 *"70% of the variation in people's weights"*: Gina Kolata, *Rethinking Thin: The New Science of Weight Loss — and the Myths and Realities of Dieting* (New York: Picador/Farrar, Straus and Giroux, 2007), 123.

145 *Keep goals few in number*: This list is adapted from Michael Hyatt, "The Beginner's Guide to Goal Setting," Michael Hyatt website, accessed June 14, 2013, http://michaelhyatt.com/goal-setting.html. See also Hyatt's book *Platform: Get Noticed in a Noisy World*.

146 *Believe and have faith in the process*: The list is adapted from Bradley Foster, "10 Steps to Successful Goal Setting," *Huffington Post*, May 7, 2013, www.huffington post.com/bradley-foster/how-to-set-goals_b_3226083.html.

149 *several reasons why making commitments doesn't work*: Leslie L. Downing, "Fragile Realities: Conversion and Commitment in Cults and Other Powerful Groups" (unpublished manuscript, 2010).

155 *Perfectionism...is a way to keep yourself safe*: Joanna Poppink, *Healing Your Hungry Heart: Recovering from Your Eating Disorder* (San Francisco: Conari Press, 2011).

Chapter 9. Balancing Work and Play

162 *play "is a state of being that is intensely pleasurable"*: "What Is Play," National Institute for Play, archived at http://archive.today/vcMgC, accessed July 27, 2014.

172 *learn more about their "dark nights"*: Thomas Moore, *Dark Nights of the Soul: A Guide to Finding Your Way through Life's Ordeals* (New York: Dover, 2003).

Index

About the Author

Karen R. Koenig, LCSW, MEd, is a psychotherapist, educator, eating coach, and expert on the *psychology of eating* — the why and how, not the what, of it — with thirty years of experience teaching overeaters and undereaters how to eat "normally" and maintain a comfortable, healthy weight for life without dieting and deprivation.

She is the author of five books: *Starting Monday, Nice Girls Finish Fat, What Every Therapist Needs to Know about Treating Eating and Weight Issues, The Food and Feelings Workbook,* and *The Rules of "Normal" Eating.* Three of her books are available in multiple foreign languages.

Her articles and essays have appeared in *Social Work Focus, Social Work Today, Eating Disorders Today,* the *Boston Globe,* the *Boston Herald,* and the *Sarasota-Herald Tribune.* She has been quoted in *Ladies Home Journal, Berner Zeitung,* the *Wall Street Journal, Women's Health, Self, Shape, Weight Watchers, In Touch,* and *OK* magazines. She has been interviewed on TV networks and programs including ABC, FOX, WHDH, SNN (Brookline, Massachusetts), and Manatee, Florida, cable, as well as on scores of radio and internet shows and podcasts.

Among other venues, she has taught seminars for Simmons College School of Social Work, Boston University School of Social Work, Massachusetts School of Professional Psychology, National Association of Social Work (Massachusetts and Florida), Massachusetts Dietetic

Association, National Organization for Women, Girl Scouts of America, and the Breast Cancer Awareness Association of Minnesota.

A graduate of Simmons College School of Social Work, Koenig practices and teaches in Sarasota, Florida. She blogs weekly at www.eating disordersblogs.com, and her website is www.karenrkoenig.com.